Cannabis Therapy

"Wendy Read has dedicated a lifetime to studying and harnessing the healing power of cannabis. Over the decades, many have had the privilege of studying with her. Now, she generously imparts her extensive knowledge and experience on the printed page. It's challenging to overestimate the importance of this publication in the field of cannabis studies; it will undoubtedly be an essential contribution for decades to come."

MATTHEW WOOD, AUTHOR OF *A SHAMANIC HERBAL* AND
HOLISTIC MEDICINE AND THE EXTRACELLULAR MATRIX

"The medicine I learned to make from Wendy has helped people overcome skin and prostate cancers and has brought health and hope to the lives of several others. Utilizing history, science, and decades of personal experience, Wendy Read presents a tome that is guaranteed to initiate the reader into a deeper relationship with cannabis for health and spiritual benefits."

CHRIS BENNETT, CANNABIS CULTIVATOR AND AUTHOR OF
CANNABIS: LOST SACRAMENT OF THE ANCIENT WORLD AND
LIBER 420: CANNABIS, MAGICKAL HERBS AND THE OCCULT

"*Cannabis Therapy: A Complete Guide* provides practitioners with a comprehensive overview of the benefits and practical applications of the herb. Wendy shares her knowledge with humor, illustrating the history and advantages of cannabis and its connection to health care. Medicinal attributes are thoroughly reviewed, and Wendy goes on to offer safe, affordable, and easy-to-make recipes for both food and medicine. Crafting your own medicine guarantees quality. Under Wendy's guidance, I have transitioned from being a client to a student and now a practitioner. The information she provides is ideal in assisting health providers and patients in navigating the benefits of marijuana for treating various issues. *Cannabis Therapy* is a beneficial resource for all cannabis practitioners."

WILLIAM R. WELLBORN, PH.D.,
PSYCHOLOGIST AND CLINICAL SPECIALIST

Cannabis Therapy

A COMPLETE GUIDE

A Sacred Planet Book

Wendy Read

Park Street Press
Rochester, Vermont

Park Street Press
One Park Street
Rochester, Vermont 05767
www.ParkStPress.com

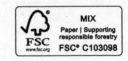

Park Street Press is a division of Inner Traditions International

Sacred Planet Books are curated by Richard Grossinger, Inner Traditions editorial board member and cofounder and former publisher of North Atlantic Books. The Sacred Planet collection, published under the umbrella of the Inner Traditions family of imprints, includes works on the themes of consciousness, cosmology, alternative medicine, dreams, climate, permaculture, alchemy, shamanic studies, oracles, astrology, crystals, hyperobjects, locutions, and subtle bodies.

Note to the reader: This book is intended to be an informational guide. The remedies, approaches, and techniques described herein are meant to supplement, and not to be a substitute for, professional medical care or treatment. They should not be used to treat a serious ailment without prior consultation with a qualified health care professional.

Cataloging-in-Publication Data for this title is available from the Library of Congress

ISBN 978-1-64411-850-4 (print)
ISBN 978-1-64411-851-1 (ebook)

Printed and bound in the United States by Lake Book Manufacturing, LLC

10 9 8 7 6 5 4 3 2 1

Text design and layout by Kenleigh Manseau
This book was typeset in Garamond Premier Pro with P22 Mackinac Pro and Soleil used as display typefaces

To send correspondence to the author of this book, mail a first-class letter to the author c/o Inner Traditions • Bear & Company, One Park Street, Rochester, VT 05767, and we will forward the communication, or contact the author directly at **caliheal.org**.

Scan the QR code and save 25% at InnerTraditions.com.
Browse over 2,000 titles on spirituality, the occult, ancient mysteries, new science, holistic health, and natural medicine.

*I dedicate this book to all those who
have been persecuted or judged for using cannabis
and to all those who seek to heal themselves and others
with this herb.*

A Note to Readers

Marijuana has been known by many names by many people. In this book I use them all with the goal of normalizing those names that have been demonized and validating the names that we have come to use and love: hemp, hashish, dagga, Mary Jane, bhang, weed, grass, cannabis, ganja, pot, mota, dope, reefer, and herb.

Contents

My Introduction to the Healing Power of Plants

All things which are old are not necessarily true; all things which are new are not necessarily without fault. To the wise men, both of them should be acceptable only if they stand to the test.

KALIDASA, HINDU POET,
C. FOURTH TO FIFTH CENTURY CE

GUATEMALA

I was living with a family in a tiny Mayan village on beautiful Lake Atitlán in Guatemala. I was studying Spanish, teaching English, and helping the local curandera, Maria, collect herbs from the base of the volcano that was her back garden. One day I was on the terrace of her cement-block home doing dishes with a green bar of soap in the outdoor sink when a young girl in a colorful handwoven traditional dress gracefully slipped by me. Inside I heard her whispering urgently to the old curandera, telling her to come quickly, her sister was bleeding. Maria grabbed her basket of herbs that was always at her side and called to me in Spanish to bring six roses from the garden. "How sweet of her to bring the family flowers in their time of need," I thought, amazed at her

1

quick thinking. I picked six roses using the hem of my skirt as protection from the thorns, and I quickly followed her through the village.

Upon arrival, she was ushered into a room separated only by a hanging blanket. I waited outside. After some low discussion and an occasional deep moan, she came back out and took me to the kitchen. There she pulled a mortar out of her basket and a few dried herbs. She began to hammer the herbs with her pestle and told me that the young woman had just given birth and was bleeding profusely and we must stop the bleeding. Then she began muttering prayers in Tz'utujil, the local Mayan language, as she continued to pound the herbs to a powder. "Hot water! Bring it, Wendy, and the roses!" I did as she said. She moistened the herbs in the mortar and added the fresh rose petals. A little more of the hot water, and then she had a pulpy, slimy mass of herbs. "Bring this and the hot water and the candle into the room. I am going for some copal." She entered the room soon after and proceeded to light a candle and burn the copal incense. Her patient was quiet and still on the bed. She was very pale, but still conscious. Another woman was busy replacing bloody pads and sheets with new ones. Maria knelt down and gently began to pack the new mother's birth canal with about half of her herbal poultice. Then she sat back and resumed praying, holding the hand of her patient and whispering prayers over her wrist. We waited. After about three minutes, blood began to seep out again. Maria gently removed the poultice and wrapped it in a cloth to hand to the other woman. She then packed the rest of the poultice in the woman's vagina. She called for a spoon, then gently fed the remaining liquid in the mortar to her patient. We waited. After five minutes, the patient's breathing calmed and deepened. After five more minutes, there was still no more seepage. The whole room took a collective deep sigh.

The herbs she used in the poultice? A local lichen, blackberry root, rose petals, and marijuana. Antiseptic, analgesic, calming, absorbent, and most of all styptic (used to stop bleeding). And copal incense to cleanse the room of *malos espíritus* and infectious germs. It worked. Her patient healed with no infection and was up and caring for her new infant within three weeks.

SCIENCE AND SPIRITUALITY

Long before I experienced spirituality, I was drawn into the world of science through a love of nature. I wanted to understand that elusive spark of life in the animals I raised, and where it went when they died. I studied biology throughout high school and college, but I was very disappointed in the cold, grey classrooms and labs as they were devoid of the life I yearned to investigate.

I did learn a lot about energy: how it was never created or destroyed, how to change it from one phase to another, and how to harness it to "do work." I learned how energy was captured when chemicals bonded and was released when they broke apart. I memorized how cells produce, store, and release energy, and how to mathematically deduce kinetic energy from potential energy. I learned that electrons are solid particles orbiting a nucleus made of other solid particles called protons and neutrons. Atoms bonded together to form molecules, and molecules were the building blocks of life. But how did a mess of molecules become infused with life? What really drove those chemical reactions? What was energy? Where was that power of life that courses through and connects everything in the universe?

Throughout my education, I was told that science was truth above all other truths and that it was the only valid system with which to heal. All others were superstition and heresy. A brief look at history told me differently. The roots of Western science come from pre-twelfth-century Europe when science and nature (spirituality) were considered two sides of the same coin. Like in indigenous cultures throughout the world, plants were sacred and people sought knowledge from them. They provided more than food, fiber, and medicine. They were respected and worshiped. Then came the newly powerful Christian church, which made science and medicine its enemy. In a colossal centuries-long land and power grab, the church murdered untold thousands of scientists, herbalists, and even cats. This ushered in the Dark Ages, when countless millions died from rodent-spread plagues, inquisitions, and ignorance. By the time Western science reemerged during the Enlightenment, it was completely divorced from spirituality and had reduced the world into people, inferior life-forms, and resources to plunder for profit. No one except for white, (mostly) male humans were accorded intelligence, respect, or a soul.

By the time I graduated in 1992, remnants of the Dark Ages still ruled scientific theory, and biology—the "study of life"—had lost its reverence for life. Without that respect, medical research (still!) often involves animal torture, the effects of which are not taken into consideration. I am appalled and deeply saddened that scientists continue to torture animals in the name of research, including research on cannabis. It is entirely safe for willing humans to experiment on themselves with cannabis. It is difficult and heartbreaking for me to review research reports that involve torture, and I heal from it by offering prayers for the animals and for the torturers, too. (I would invite the reader to do so as well, because group prayer is always more powerful.)

I do watch hopefully these days as science once again begins to wonder at the invisible, energetic, and spiritual aspects of nature. Physicists demonstrate that what they once thought were particles of matter are really waves of energy that only condense into matter when being observed. Does that mean that all solid matter on Earth is being observed? Is this not a spiritual question? Biologists today now consider *ecosystems* instead of *organisms* because they are learning that organisms within a system are connected and cannot thrive without each other. Beyond the chemical makeup of a single plant, chemists study the complex communication channels that fill a forest floor with great webs of mycelium. Medical science no longer ignores the digestive system when studying the heart or the nervous system when studying digestion. When they are ignorant of the function of an organ, like the appendix, or strands of DNA outside of the double helix, they no longer label them as junk.

Science is on the threshold of having to reform its foundational structure. If mere observation affects the outcome of an experiment, then "impartial," "controlled," and "double-blind" experimentation, the foundation of scientific method, is impossible. For accurate interpretations of results, we must consider innumerable, uncontrollable, and even unknown parameters. What are the energetic effects imposed by the observer? What was the emotional condition of the tortured rat? What are the effects of past trauma on the physiology of a test subject given a placebo? Our perspective must widen to include even things like the position of the moon and stars in the cosmos.

The false dichotomy of Western science and spirituality has taught us the dangers of blind, singular faith in either. Science should not be embraced with blind faith, nor considered a "savior." Nor should faith be adhered to blindly without the support of scientific principles. Together, however, they are the most powerful way to experience the world around us. I hope to see science rediscover the obvious—that all life has a spiritual component, and each life is a complex strand interwoven in a multidimensional, invisible, immeasurable web of energy. To tweak a strand sends invisible vibrations through the whole web.

And so after earning degrees in biology and chemistry in the early 1990s, I forsook the corporate jobs and advanced degrees available to me, and I opted instead for self-satisfying and self-driven education through travel and reading. I specifically sought out teachers and tribes that lived with the Earth, healed themselves with her herbs, and connected with her through ritual. I studied with and continue to learn from the ultimate teacher, Mother Nature herself.

ON TO AFRICA

As I stumbled out of that dark room in Guatemala and into the hot sunlight, I was once again awed by my surroundings. The lake radiated peace. The high, oh-so-steep mountain peaks surrounding it shimmered and danced with ancient power, and I could almost sense tremors coming up from the caldera with no bottom. Timeless. Well, almost.

With the excitement I had almost forgotten what day it was. Now I must hurry in this unhurried land, for I had a very important appointment to keep . . .

A Maya fisherman was poling his boat close to the shore. I waved him over and asked for a ride across the lake. Stepping into the wooden, hand-carved, flat-bottom canoe, a *kayuko,* I quickly sat down on the bottom. Had I stood, like the fisherman, I would have upset the delicate balance of the boat and possibly sent both of us into the water. Upon return visits, I would learn to paddle one on my own, but today his innate skill floated us across the caldera.

I disembarked in the shallows and stumbled onto dry land with my flip-flops in my hand. There was no time to stop and chat with the market ladies lining the path as I climbed the steep rise to the phone office. Perhaps if you traveled internationally in the '70s or '80s you came upon a phone office. This one was a small cement-block building with a low ceiling. Inside were three cabinets that looked like phone booths, each with a chair and a low table supporting a heavy, black, round-dialed phone. I approached the Maya man behind the counter and spoke with him in my rudimentary Spanish—a second language for both of us. I handed him the crumpled piece of torn paper I'd pulled from the secret pocket I wore under my skirt. He read the address and phone number I had written on it many months ago, just before leaving the states for this current adventure.

"Washington? Washington, DC?" He shouted with delight.

"Clinton? You get call from Clinton?" he asked, looking up from the paper. A row of perfect white teeth flashed at me from the broad smile that took over his round face.

"Well, not exactly . . ." I replied, at a loss to explain the complicated nature of the call in my basic Spanish.

"OK, OK, OK, senorita, please, you sit. I call Clinton!" Laughing, he turned away to complete the difficult business of placing an international call. I chose the chair with only one metal coil springing up from the cracked green Naugahyde seat.

Forty sweaty, fly-filled minutes later he shouted my name and that of my president across the tiny room, capturing the interest of the others waiting silently in the office. The businessman with the pink Scooby-Doo backpack turned toward me curiously, as did the grandmother, whose colorfully striped, handwoven full skirt perfectly complimented her yellow and green Mickey Mouse T-shirt.

What I heard was, "Wendy, Clinton, ooo-neet-ade stat-is piss coo for you. Cabin Three." His delight elevated his chuckle to a roar as he turned to an old metal filing cabinet that screeched its horror at being rudely jerked open.

I barely fit inside the phone cabin—Guatemala being built for people of small stature—but I managed and had just closed the accordion door with a few awkward jerks when the phone coughed up a shrill ring. It had been so long since I had heard that sound, and I was so nervous, that for a minute I just stared at the coiled cord attached like a snake to the heavy base as if I were an alien Yip Yip from Sesame Street. It rang again. This time I managed to lift the receiver and say hello.

I could barely understand the woman on the other end through the severe crackling on the line. I was suddenly paranoid that we would be cut off before I heard the news I had called to hear.

"Congratulations, Miss ***-heim. We have *** United States Peace Corps assignment. You will be placed in Sw***z**land."

"Uh, thank you. Switzerland? There is Peace Corps in Switzerland?"

"No ma'am, Sw***z**land. S-w-a-z-i-l-a-n-d," she spelled out carefully.

"Oh. Great. I mean . . . where exactly is that?"

"Swaziland is a small landlocked kingdom in Africa."

"Africa? You're sending me to Africa? But I speak Spanish . . ."

"This is your current assignment. You have the right to turn it down and we will find you another, but you will be put at the bottom of the list."

"No! I'm game! I've been waiting for this for months! Is it, uh, an agricultural assignment? Or related to my science degree?"

"In a way . . . it looks like you will be a teacher . . . I really don't have any more details than that. Oh, and you need to report to Philadelphia on July 28th. If you have any more questions, please contact our training office. Congratulations again, and good luck." She cheerily rang off, after changing my life forever.

July 28? That meant that I had about three weeks to get to Pennsylvania, and I first had to travel by bus across the giant country of Mexico and back to California. But first things first, I spent the evening searching the village for a map of the world. Would you believe it was conveniently located in a bar?

We were lucky and very spoiled in the tiny country of Swaziland in 1993 (now called by its native name, Eswatini). Most of us Peace Corps volunteers were within a few hours of towns, and our decorated and comically christened buses, like "In God's Hands" or "Impact Bus Service," only broke down semiregularly. We also learned that we could safely hitchhike anywhere in the Southern Africa region.

I decided to try this out early on—this hitchhiking system that the old volunteers had taught us, and that all the Swazis used. I threw on my second skin—my backpack—walked a ways to the main road and waved my right palm down toward the road with my left hand placed firmly on my right elbow. (One always displayed the left hand this way. As in many cultures, it was traditionally used as toilet paper and was never offered to another. This included waving, shaking hands, transactions with money, and hitchhiking. To this day, I still find myself performing this action on occasion from habit.)

Almost immediately an old bearded *babe* (meaning "father," pronounced "bah-beh") pulled over with a grin in his ancient British backy (pickup truck), which was once painted turquoise. When I greeted him in siSwati, he became very excited and enthusiastic as he drove us on down the road. After the greetings and patter died out naturally, I sat back to enjoy the breathtaking scenery of the mountainous "high veld" area of Eswatini.

Before long, however, he picked up a piece of seemingly stray newspaper and placed it carefully over his lap. He began fiddling in his crotch. "Well fuck," I thought. "Here we go! Count on me to catch my first ride with one of those!" I pointedly stared out my window and began looking for a safe place to disembark from this now uncomfortable ride. The passenger door was not locked, and if he refused to pull over, I figured I could jump out around a slow curve if I had to. But before I could contemplate my escape further, the rustling in his lap ceased. I chanced a quick look just as he proudly held up—the biggest cigarette I had ever seen! I don't think I contained my sigh of relief.

It wasn't tobacco, either. He promptly lit the pachyderm-size reefer, took a great inhale as he turned to face me, and offered it with a slow smile. I looked in his eyes and realized that I was in no danger. I still declined, though, as I was brand new in the village and knew that news would travel fast if I partook. My reply, "No thank you, Babe," was greeted with a nod. He took one more hit of his giant news-wrapped joint, and then he just threw the rest out of the window. "Holy shit," I remember thinking, "I'm gonna like living here!"

HIDDEN NATURE

For the next four years, I lived in and traveled throughout Africa. After finishing with my Peace Corps assignment, I traveled throughout the Southern Africa region and then explored Morocco, Mauritania, Mali, and Senegal. I spent a lot of time in England on layovers. At one point I stayed with a friend for a month in Birmingham. She was a physician and I learned a lot from her by accompanying her on her house calls. When I ran low on money, I would return to work for short stints in California to fund the next leg of my journey. I was able to offer basic first aid in most of the villages I stayed in, and I connected with as many traditional healers as I could, learning about their herbal medicines and tribal rituals.

As a radical American, I found I had to grapple with how much of "me" to keep hidden from the different tribal communities I visited and lived with. I changed my dress, my posture, my diet, how I spoke, how I worshiped, and much more. I held back stories from my life and plans for my future. I gave up all privacy except in the outhouse. As a single white woman living with black or brown tribes, I was in a fishbowl, the object of stares, frequent marriage proposals, and curious company wherever I was, all the time. Since white women in Southern Africa (and often in Central America) never set foot in black or indigenous villages, rode buses, or shopped in the outdoor markets, I was quite a shock for most villagers. In Eswatini, the always-crowded communal water tap was right outside my window, and windows were there for peeking through. In a tribe where most girls gave birth in their teens to show that they were marriable, Swazis could not believe that I was unmarried and had no children. I found myself always on guard to hide my true, wild, adventurous self. I was constantly afraid that I would offend by accident with a misdeed or the wrong word.

In Eswatini I lived and taught at a Christian school. Most Swazis practice a conservative Christianity called Zionism. I just could not force myself to spend entire days or evenings sitting on church pews with them, so I took these times to commune in nature my own way, which often included smoking dagga, or pot. I hid my interest in traditional medicine from my friends while I secretly sought out Southern African shamans, called *sangomas* or *inyangas*. They were themselves publicly ostracized but discreetly visited by "modern" Christian Swazis. The soccer coach would bring his team for a blessing before games, or villagers would secretly come to have curses removed or ailments cured.

Behaviors completely against my culture's morals and values were not only accepted by Swazis but embedded in their culture, and I had to learn to withhold my judgments and hide my shock. Stealing was accepted and endemic. My fellow teachers would steal things like staplers from my desk and then proudly tell me about it the next day. Without dishonor or shame for either party, teachers impregnated their teenage students, who then had to drop out of school. It seemed commonplace to hear that someone had been purposely poisoned to death: "Oh, so-and-so is sick. He was poisoned by his coworker. He is in hospital now and will not live."

Initially I wanted to "fix" those seemingly horrendous situations according to my own ethics. I viewed their culture as a failed attempt at living like mine. When I could get away, I would hike in the hills, smoke some dagga, and get the cattle egrets' perspective as they soared over the valley. This helped me immensely to process day-to-day living in a very foreign culture.

Eventually, with more world experience and altered perspectives courtesy of marijuana, I learned many great spiritual lessons and tackled the innate racism in myself. I came to realize that my culture was not superior to others, and other cultures were not a failed attempt at living mine. Every culture is valid and beautiful and every human is doing the best they can according to the circumstances they were born into. If a person or a culture is cut off from nature, or their own true nature, they will sicken.

Hiding my true self was a survival skill that suited my life in tribal cultures. I balanced the difficulties by connecting with nature. Much later, as I began my work as a healer, I came to understand that when people are forced to protect themselves by hiding their true nature or emotions from their innermost circle of friends, coworkers, or family, it can have a devastating effect on their health, unless they can balance that out with a strong connection to their own soul. Mary Jane is always here to help me maintain that connection.

THE EMERALD TRIANGLE

More than five years and countless adventures later, I returned to the states. I found a strong, land-based community in Northern California, settled down, and found home. Due to its underground lifestyle, it took me a year to discover I was in the heart of the Emerald Triangle. This tricounty region is infamous for producing the highest quality buds in the world and providing them to the rest of the country. The Pacific Northwest is also chock-full of radical activists, herbalists, and natural healers. I could not have designed a better place to live for myself.

I began cultivating weed under the guidance of my best friend and mentor, Brother Bruce. I found local teachers and began an in-depth study of the healing arts. I was living alone, caretaking a 160-acre off-grid horse ranch. It was five miles up a dirt road on a 3,300-foot mountain, one hour from the mystical Mendocino coast. My apartment was on top of a giant barn with an amazing 360-degree view of the redwood- and oakwood-covered mountains and the river valley below. There was a phone on a "farm line" in the barn below that I rarely used, and which didn't work in the rainy season. It was a psychically powerful spot, and I began receiving strong visions connected to my own healing and future work. After three years, the place sold and I moved down into the valley and continued to practice massage therapy, energy healing, and gardening.

One day I was out in my pot patch enjoying a sunny day. I heard a deep voice behind me say, "You know, you could be growing a lot of other herbs out here. . ." Startled out of my solitude, I literally looked around for the source. It was coming from the pot patch! Well, of course plants can talk, I laughed to myself, remembering all the shamans and witches I had encountered during my travels. Three days later, a friend handed me a flyer for a women's herbal school called Motherland. I dove in and completed a nine-month course together with thirteen other women. After graduating I continued my studies, began making medicine in earnest, and started teaching at Motherland, local herbal symposiums, and other herb schools. I continued to seek out teachers in the healing arts and attended classes all over the Pacific Northwest in massage therapy, energy healing, and herbal medicine. I was lucky to discover an experienced clinical practitioner of plant-spirit healing and apprenticed with her for a year in California and Vermont.

In most of my classes I would ask the teacher what they thought about the healing properties of marijuana. Without fail every one told me that there were none, or that there were other herbs that were far better. The most experienced and educated herbalists in the country were completely sure, and sometimes obstinate, that pot caused more harm than good.

HOLISTIC HEALING

As it is not proper to try to cure the eyes without the head, nor the head without the body, so neither is it proper to cure the body without the soul, and this is the reason why so many diseases escape physicians who are ignorant of the whole.

PLATO, *CHARMIDES, OR TEMPERANCE*

Having come full circle in my search to understand energy, I was now able to experience life's energy directly in plants, animals, and people, and to manipulate it for healing using my hands and my heart. Through my studies in ayurveda and traditional Chinese medicine, I had learned that energy must flow freely through all beings for health, and disruption in the flow can lead to imbalance and dis-ease. Dis-ease in one part of an organism affects the whole organism. Poison one organism and you poison the whole ecosystem, including yourself. The death of any ecosystem leads to the death of all the ecosystems. Conversely, strengthening an organism strengthens its ecosystem, yourself, and the Earth. This is the philosophy behind holistic healing and this is why I call myself a holistic healer.

Whereas allopathic medicine views symptoms of dis-ease as illnesses to be suppressed, holistic healers see them as messengers of imbalance that direct a healer and client to look deeper for the cause. Chemotherapy, for instance, is carcinogenic. It may shrink a cancerous tumor in an organism, but will also cause great harm that radiates out from the patient. These toxic chemicals are not broken down by the organism and they continue on to pollute the water system, causing more disease in the greater environment. They can also cause later cancer in the user—especially if the patient doesn't rectify the underlying imbalances that caused the cancer to erupt.

Holistic health practitioners might provide treatment for symptom relief, but only as an adjunct to correcting the underlying causes. Holistic treatments do not cause harm to the client or the environment. These therapies encompass a multitude of natural, harmless modalities that address the mind, body, and spirit of an organism. In my case they include many forms of massage therapy, energy healing, spiritual counseling, visualization, trance work, herbal medicine, and shamanic healing techniques. This broad array allows me to blend appropriate modalities into unique therapies designed to resonate with each individual client.

An Example of a Holistic Treatment for Someone Suffering from Anxiety

Start with 1 steaming bath

(Relaxes muscles, stimulates circulation)

Add 2 cups Epsom salts

(Draw out toxins and bruising, supplements magnesium, relaxes muscles)

Add 3 drops of lavender essential oil

(Calming, uplifting, antimicrobial, soothes sore muscles, encourages deep breathing)

Add 1 bath bag with cannabis leaves and chamomile

(Anti-inflammatory, calming)

Add 3 drops of the flower essence of your choice

(Balances emotions, connects you with your spirit)

Light 1 candle

(Focal point to clear the mind)

Play music of your choice: calming, inspirational, trance inducing, or songs you like to sing aloud

(Changes brain waves, clears the mind)

Repeat as necessary

Early in my practice I came to realize that many issues my clients suffered from were rooted in spiritual disconnection. Again and again, buried behind complaints of exhaustion, depression, anxiety, chronic pain, digestive disorders, and more, I find deeper spiritual issues like unprocessed grief, bottled-up emotions, repressed memories, unhealed past traumas, or current or past abuse. On top of that, multilayered issues are often aggravated by an unconscious attempt to ignore them. People fall prey to patterns of addiction, eating disorders, interpersonal drama, risky behavior, abusing others, or hiding in victimhood to provide distraction from—or some semblance of control over—deeper problems that they feel helpless to address. Realizing this, I began offering seasonal rituals eight times a year for my community that helped them (and me) develop spiritual practices to improve our well-being.

THE EMERALD TRINITY

The power of the experiences, thoughts, and perspectives intertwined in our bodies never ceases to fascinate me. Our issues live in our tissues, and when our spirits are stifled, our bodies suffer. Problems with spiritual health affect our physical health, just as a chronic physical condition can cause mental illness. Because Mary Jane can heal the mind, body, and spirit, she calls herself the Emerald Trinity. Because Mary Jane has a mind, body, and spirit, I call her that as well.

But how does the suppression of something as intangible as memories or feelings lead to bodily distress? How does fear cause us to perspire and tremble, or love make us laugh or tear up? How does changing these intangibles change our bodies? And how does marijuana effect this trinity of connections?

This is where my love of mysticism and medicine meet. I am fascinated by the multidimensional energetic cords that connect our thoughts, feelings, and behaviors to our somatic chemicals and solid muscles. Our physical, mental, and spiritual functions are so deeply interwoven at the biochemical level that they cannot be healed separately. A laugh can strengthen your heart, an insult can change the color of your face. Your laugh can strengthen someone else's heart. Your insult can change the color of someone else's face. How far into the universe do these vibrations spread? Where are the bridges that connect our spirits to our molecular chemistry?

I discovered one such bridge in our endocannabinoid system (ECS). The ECS, found not just in humans but in all animals, is a foundational part of the web of life, and it is our direct connection to marijuana. Chemicals produced by both animal cells and the cannabis plant direct the dance of molecules inside us that inspire action and modify behavior. The endocannabinoid system integrates all our psychic, spiritual, and somatic functions. (And those of your little dog, too!) The ECS is the link between your body, mind, and spirit, and it is the foundational structure providing the near miraculous effects of the Emerald Trinity.

HOW TO USE THIS BOOK

The first chapters of this book share basic knowledge about marijuana medicine. Chapter 1 explores the endocannabinoid system and its interaction with cannabis in detail. Chapter 2 reconciles the myths and confusion around the herb that stem from a long history of persecution, demonization, and propaganda by shedding light on the truth.

Chapter 3, "Whole Plant Medicine," shares a list of herbal actions followed by a review of the known medicinal plant constituents and their locations in the plant, from her crown to her roots. In chapter 4 I break through many barriers by showing how getting high is actually *good* for your health and mental well-being. Chapter 5 describes how cannabis functions within each body system and explains why she helps to cure such a diverse spectrum of illnesses and injuries—from broken bones to gut issues to cancer to COVID. A list of general symptoms that weed can relieve is given as well.

In chapter 6 I provide a comprehensive list of marijuana medicines and describe for each medicine its time of onset, duration of effect, risk of THC overdose, target areas of the body, and conditions that each medicine is ideal for. Here you will find a useful table ranking the psychoactivity ranges for various THC medicines and you will also find treatments for an overdose of THC. Chapter 7 discusses how to incorporate cannabis into other healing methods such as massage, breathwork, flower essences, aromatherapy, diet, exercise, rest, and meditation.

Chapter 8 brings all previous information together to help the reader design a marijuana therapy plan for themselves or others. I offer guidance on how to develop a plan, how to evaluate its effects, and how to adapt it as you go, including many illustrative case stories.

Chapter 9 is a do-it-yourself guide for beginners who want to make simple marijuana medicines. I have included delicious recipes with raw weed, hemp seeds, and hemp seed oil, as well as detailed instructions for making teas, tinctures, liniments, infused oils, salves, aromatherapy medicines, and more. Experienced medicine makers can take these basic medicines and formulate them into more complex remedies.

Chapter 10 is for those who want to use ganja spiritually or to help others heal their spirits. Here you will discover how your ancestors imbibed, and how many of the great spiritualities and religions of the world grew from her sacred seed.

For thirty-four years I have studied holistic healing from curanderas in Mexico, Maya shamans in Guatemala, sangomas in Eswatini, and grandmothers and masters throughout the world. I have cultivated and made medicine from marijuana and hundreds of different medicinal herbs for the past twenty years. I've led a pagan church and maintained a holistic clinical practice for fifteen years. I am an herbalist, massage therapist, priestess, shaman, medicine maker, spiritual counselor, and teacher.

Now I want to reach beyond my students, congregation, and clients. I want to share my knowledge of marijuana medicine with a larger world that is increasingly ready to receive it. As states and countries all over the globe are coming to accept this deeply medicinal plant and legislate her back into freedom, I want to help the people find her and bring her back into their lives. Together we can elevate the Queen of Herbs back to her rightful place as the greatest of human allies and the foundation of balance for our health and our planet.

So, I ask you, reader, to bring an open heart, an open mind, and an appreciation for both science and spirituality to these pages as we explore marijuana and her world, the essence of the Emerald Trinity.

1

Cannabinoids and the Endocannabinoid System

Before we can contemplate marijuana as medicine, we need to understand the complex endocannabinoid system (ECS). The ECS, found in all animals, is the physical avenue by which marijuana interacts with our bodies, our minds, and our spirits, writing the codes for health and bliss.

The story of the ECS begins 34 million years ago when life as we know it began in the great Mother Ocean. The first beings, enclosed in a single cell, were free-floating and self-contained. They could not survive alone, however. Like us, they needed communication with others to thrive. Even at the beginning all life was connected, albeit with invisible threads, in a magnificent energetic web.

Exactly how were those cells talking with each other as they were propelled through the chaotic tides? They were sending and receiving tiny packets of chemicals produced within their membranes.

Can you imagine each cell opening its doors to receive news brought on the current, like a housewife welcoming gossip from a door-to-door fruit seller? Possibly the updates were about the usual things, like the weather or where to find favorite foods. Perhaps they, too, warned each other about which neighborhoods to avoid due to unfavorable conditions or unsavory characters. And the chemical messages themselves? They were cannabinoids, or more accurately, phospholipid cannabinoid precursors.

When I ask my students what a cannabinoid is, few can answer. But when I ask for an example of a cannabinoid, inevitably they shout out "THC!" Short for tetrahydrocannabinol, THC is the most famous cannabinoid in the world. THC is a phytocannabinoid, created by a plant, rather than an endocannabinoid, which are created by animals. The two kinds of cannabinoids have slightly different structures, but share many functions within an animal system.

Today's cannabinoids are still tiny, comprised of a molecular chain of a mere twenty-two to twenty-five carbon atoms. Cannabinoids' main function is to carry directions and information between animal cells. They are often classified as neurotransmitters because they send signals through and between the nerve cells that make up the nervous system. Neurotransmitters, including serotonin and dopamine, the cannabinoids' more famous cousins, are well-known for the powerful role they play within the body and mind. For example, pharmaceutical antidepressants called serotonin reuptake inhibitors, or SSRIs, change the way our bodies process serotonin. As anyone who has used them can attest, their effects on the body and the emotions can be extreme. The feeling a mother has when cradling her infant is the work of oxytocin, another neurotransmitter. That feeling of well-being some experience when eating chocolate and the devastatingly intense grief when a loved one dies are both a result of neurotransmitters.

As it turns out, cannabinoids control the nervous system. In addition to a multitude of other duties, they rule over the other neurotransmitters. For example, cannabinoids indirectly increase dopamine levels by blocking the action of another neurotransmitter, GABA, which reduces the amount of dopamine released. When GABA is blocked by marijuana compounds, the result is an increase in the amount of dopamine released. Cannabis is nature's answer to SSRIs, but unlike SSRIs, she follows the edict "First, do no harm" and brings the body into balance without unhealthy side effects or withdrawal symptoms.

How did we get to the complex ECS from those primordial single-celled beings? As those cells were floating around, they would bump into each other, perhaps even seeking each other out. At some point, they started to realize the advantages of floating through life together and decided to form colonies. They drifted around like little rafts, with those in the middle well protected from outside influences like viruses and other predators, and those on the edges having first access to food. When some cells perished, cannabinoid signals were sent out, triggering others to divide into two daughter cells, thus replenishing the colony.

Eventually, for protection, some colonies surrounded themselves with a membrane and became, in essence, a gated community. Cells worked together and consciously chose what entered and what exited, essentially taking in groceries and sending out the garbage. Just as a baker or weaver provides a specific service to the village, cells within the colony began to specialize and differentiate from one another by turning on only a small section, or sequence, within their protein-producing DNA. Some turned into skin cells, others feather cells, others became brain cells, and so forth. They continued to use cannabinoids to communicate.

All animals produce cannabinoids that control life's functions. Created on demand, they leap between the axon of one nerve to the dendrite of the next. They float through our blood until a cell fishes them out of the slipstream and pulls them inside. There, the cannabinoids deliver direction to stimulate or (more often) inhibit the cell's function, speeding or slowing, starting or stopping pathways of creation or courses of destruction. Together, these millions of tiny alterations throughout our systems continually guide us toward homeostasis, trying to keep us in balance.

Just as we raise a flag on our mailbox to signal outgoing mail, cells throw up a flag on the outside of their membranes when they need to take in nutrients, expel waste, or receive directions for their work. These flags, aptly named receptors, are the fishhooks, and they are baited to attract only a specific kind of chemical from the stream. Once caught, a porthole in the cell membrane opens, and the cannabinoid or other chemical is reeled in.

THE BLISS MOLECULE

Certain "magical" plants, animals, and funguses have always provided spiritual healing to animals. The witches, prophets, and seers of indigenous spiritualities have ancient relationships with beings like peyote cacti, psilocybin mushrooms, herbs like ayahuasca and ibogaine, and many others. These beings help them heal themselves and others by connecting them with the invisible world of energy that surrounds us. On a deep level, humans have always known about the magical effects of marijuana. Unfortunately, these magical substances have been demonized by cultural authorities and driven underground off and on for thousands of years. At this time in history, many are coming back into the light and are beginning to pique the interest of Western medicine.

Take, for example, the opium poppy. Used in Asia for thousands of years and brought to the West during the mid-nineteenth century Opium Wars between China and England, this delicate flower has one of the strongest known pain-relieving effects in the world, and she also provides a spiritual sense of well-being. In the 1970s Western scientists became curious about how she works in our system. With new technology they were able to isolate opium molecules and mark them with a radioactive dye. When injected into an animal, they could see them course through an animal's system and note where they were absorbed. They discovered and mapped the system of opium receptors in animals.[1]

But why do animals, for which poppies are not a food source, produce pain reduction receptor sites specific for opium molecules? Continuing investigations revealed that these receptors are actually designed to capture opium molecules produced by the animals themselves.

Called endorphins (from *endogenous* meaning "produced within" and *morphine,* a pain-relieving alkaloid made by poppies), these chemicals produced by our bodies help block pain signals and offer a sense of peace and well-being. When our endorphins prove insufficient for intense pain, poppy plants act as a perfectly designed supplement. The discovery of the poppy-activated endorphin system spurred scientists to search for other systems activated by naturally occurring drugs.

Although THC was discovered in 1964 by Israeli researcher Raphael Mechoulam, Ph.D., it was not until three decades later that his team searched for endogenous THC receptors in animals. The only well-known use of weed at that time was to get people high, so they hypothesized that they would find receptors for THC in the brain. They synthesized cannabinoids, dyed them, and injected them into animals to trace their pathway. They were right about the brain, of course, but were surprised when they also found receptors throughout the entire central nervous system.

Scientists knew that the fact that THC made people high indicated that, like opium, it could cross the blood-brain barrier. The blood-brain barrier is a protective lining that surrounds the central nervous system (the CNS) and forms a strong line of defense between the blood circulating through our bodies and the fluid that circulates within the CNS. It controls what passes between the two and, for example, allows animals to endure extreme infections and other toxic insults without brain damage. Most pharmaceutical drugs, even antibiotics and cancer treatments, are too toxic to be allowed through the barrier, yet our central nervous system readily invites marijuana into its inner sanctum. This is partly why cannabis provides such a myriad of therapies for the mind.

When Mechoulam found the first endocannabinoid, meaning a cannabinoid endogenous to animals, in 1992, he demonstrated his immediate understanding of its power when he named the molecule *anandamide*. *Ananda* means "bliss" in Sanskrit, the language of the Vedas, the world's most ancient religious texts. They are dedicated to the worship of Soma, a deity, and a cannabis tea. (The full story is told in chapter 10.) Upon discovery of a second endocannabinoid, Mechoulam forsook all sense of poetry and named it 2-arachidonoyl glycerol, or 2AG for short. Since then, two more endocannabinoids, lysophosphatidylinositol and virodhamine, have been discovered, and it is safe to assume that more will be found soon.

RECEIVING BLISS

Cannabinoid receptors consist of long chains of proteins that weave back and forth through a cell membrane seven times, like magical serpents.

By acting both as flags to attract cannabinoids to a cell and sentries to open the gates, receptors in essence invite cannabis into our cells.

The receptors found throughout the brain and central nervous system are called CB1 receptors, for cannabinoid receptors type one. Cannabinoid receptors are more abundant in the brain than any other type of neurotransmitter receptor.

When CB2 receptors were first discovered in 1993, they seemed to be absent from the CNS but prolific in the peripheral nervous system and the rest of the body. The highest concentration of CB2 receptors was found in the immune system, specifically on the B lymphocytes, the white blood cells that produce antibodies. CB2 receptors are also found in the spleen, tonsils, and thymus gland. They are on hemato-poietic cells—the stem cells that give rise to all the other types of blood cells—and are also throughout the gastrointestinal system, the adipose tissue, and the reproductive system.

Later experiments found CB2 receptor sites in the CNS also, although at a much lower concentration than CB1 sites. The CB2 receptors demonstrate that marijuana medicine is invited not just into the mind, but into every part of the body.

When activated by cannabinoids, CB1 and CB2 receptors turn on anti-inflammatory effects that help relieve pain and protect animals from inflammation-driven diseases like arthritis, asthma, diabetes, and neuropathy (the painful death of nerve cells that can be triggered by diabetes and other diseases). These receptors are key in preventing and treating obesity and other metabolic disorders. They also protect against brain damage from strokes, concussions, and neurodegenerative ailments like Parkinson's disease.

The beautiful dance between cannabinoids and our bodies becomes ever more complex and graceful when a phytocannabinoid attends the ball. Together, all the cannabinoids intertwine with receptors and enzymes to either invite in more endocannabinoids and neurotransmitters or show them to the door, depending on what the situation needs to achieve balance.

Scientists continue to discover more cannabinoid receptors with different capabilities and other plant and animal chemicals that activate them. Some cannabinoids, like cannabidiol (CBD for short), don't work directly with receptors but utilize more complex, and less understood, biochemical pathways. And in addition to cannabinoids and receptors, the endocannabinoid system also includes many enzymes that catalyze the production and breakdown of these chemicals.

In the process of researching the biochemical pathway for getting high, science has learned that all vertebrate animals have an endocannabinoid system made up of internally produced cannabinoids and receptors that regulate every system of the body. The ECS can also be activated by phytocannabinoids. This knowledge has increased the power to heal exponentially.

THE ROLE OF THE ECS

The biggest killer on the planet is stress, and I still think the best medicine is and always has been cannabis.

WILLIE NELSON

In general, the ECS regulates six basic life systems: relaxing, sleeping, eating, protecting, reproducing, and forgetting. It does this in a myriad of ways within the systems of our bodies. When the ECS is struggling, sometimes called "cannabinoid deficiency syndrome," we can experience symptoms like lack of appetite, digestive difficulties, free-floating anxiety, insomnia, fatigue, oxidative stress, and an inability to focus. When the ECS is impaired, supplementing with cannabis can be extremely effective.

The ECS is responsible for balancing the two parts of our autonomous nervous system (ANS): the sympathetic nervous system, which is engaged when we are preparing for or performing an action, and the parasympathetic nervous system, which allows us to slow down, relax, sleep, get hungry, and digest our food.

A healthy ECS protects our tissues and organs from toxins, oxidative damage, chronic inflammation, and pain, thus preventing a myriad of diseases and injuries.

The ECS helps us forget. ("Aha!" I hear you say, "I knew pot was bad for my memory!" Au contraire, that is not what we mean by "forgetting.") The ECS filters out the background noise of our lives. Subconsciously, our brains continually prune sensory input out of our immediate focus, protecting us from constant overstimulation. The process of "forgetting," of editing and filtering out the visual, auditory, and memory stimulus of life, is an adaptive strategy that the human mind needs to be healthy and happy. A dysfunctional filtering system is often a symptom of autism and, for some, of schizophrenia. It can also be the death of creativity and our sense of wonder.

Forgetting or filtering is necessary for us to dishabituate, find fresh perspective, and experience peace of mind. For example, when someone is high and bites into a peach, they can think it is the most delicious peach they have ever tasted. In truth, the high has helped them "forget" about all the peaches they have tasted before so they can focus completely on the experience in the present. The ECS helps us forget by filtering out unnecessary distractions and information so that we can focus on the important things in life.

WHAT CANNABINOIDS DO

At the time of this writing, marijuana is still a Schedule I drug, defined as "having a high potential for abuse and no currently accepted medical use." Permission for research is near impossible to get in the United States. As of August 2022, only seven licenses have been issued in the United States for the manufacture of cannabis and cannabis medicines for research.[2] Why, then, did the U.S. government itself file for a patent on cannabinoid medicines in 1999? And why was the patent granted in 2003? Let's look at how much the patent reveals about the true power of marijuana medicine, what the U.S. government has known and hidden for over twenty years.[3]

The patent application claims that cannabinoids are a "treatment and prophylaxis of a wide variety of oxidation associated diseases, such as ischemic, age-related, inflammatory, and autoimmune diseases.

Cannabinoids have particular application as neuroprotectants, for example in limiting neurological damage following ischemic insults, such as stroke and trauma, or in the treatment of neurodegenerative diseases, such as Alzheimer's disease, Parkinson's disease, Down's Syndrome, and HIV dementia." Cannabinoids, the application continues, are also "useful as tissue protectants, such as neuroprotectants and cardio-protectants."

Let's break this down.

Prophylaxis means "prevention." So not only is the government acknowledging that cannabis is a treatment for many diseases but also that it can prevent them.

Cannabis is a very strong antioxidant. That is, it prevents and treats oxidative damage and the diseases that result from it. Most people have heard of antioxidants from the natural food and health industries promoting their "anti-aging" effects. Oxidative damage is caused by oxygen atoms (or molecules—a combination of atoms) with an unpaired electron that steal electrons from other atoms or molecules. An oxygen atom with an unpaired electron is called an oxidant, or a "free radical."

Free radicals are formed as part of normal metabolic processes in the cell and are usually neutralized before they can cause trouble. However, they are also formed from stress on the cell such as inflammatory reactions, toxic exposure, radiation exposure, or blunt trauma. Too many free radicals, or oxidants, will stress the repair system and cause oxidative damage by overwhelming the cleanup crew. The resultant tissue death leads to what the media calls the "signs of aging": wrinkles, dryness, grey hair, and loss of vision, cognitive function, and memory.

Antioxidants correct and prevent oxidative damage. Dietary antioxidants include vitamins C and E and the flavonoids found in red, blue, and purple fruits, red wine, and green tea. Cannabinoids are about one thousand times stronger than other antioxidants. They are able to penetrate our tissues and nervous system because cannabis is fat-soluble and can cross the fatty layer at the center of our semipermeable cell membranes—a layer that helps the cell control what enters and leaves it. Thus, they can cross the blood-brain barrier to do their prevention and cleanup work inside the brain and central nervous system, which other antioxidants cannot access.

The next medical benefit discussed in the 2003 patent application are ischemic events. Ischemia is damage to cells and tissues due to a restriction of blood supply, and therefore of oxygen and glucose. Some of the damage is due to the release of glutamate, which creates—you guessed it—free radicals. If you know anyone who has suffered a stroke or a heart attack, you have seen the effects of ischemia. Cannabis's antioxidant power can prevent such damage. In fact, as the patent application claims:

It is an object of this invention to provide a new class of antioxidant drugs that can access the brain, and are generally useful in the treatment of many oxidation associated diseases. . . . This invention provides antioxidant compounds and compositions, such as pharmaceutical compositions, that include cannabinoids that act as free radical scavengers for use in prophylaxis and treatment of disease. The invention also includes methods for using the antioxidants in prevention and treatment of pathological conditions such as ischemia and in subjects who have been exposed to oxidant inducing agents such as cancer chemotherapy, toxins, radiation, or other sources of oxidative stress. The compositions and methods described herein are also used for preventing oxidative damage in transplanted organs, for inhibiting reoxygenation injury (for example in heart disease), and for any other condition that is mediated by oxidative or free radical mechanisms of injury.[4]

Cannabis is the world's best anti-inflammatory. When the body is infected or injured it sends inflammatory cells, called cytokines, to the area. Cytokines mark the injury and attract immune cells to the area to kill and clean up the invading substance. These cells poke holes in blood cells, causing them to leak fluid at the site of the injury, and the resulting swelling and stiffness pillow and protect the injury from movement and impact so that it may heal. That is acute inflammation, a powerful defense mechanism that clears away when the area heals. The suffix -itis means "inflamed." For example, bronchitis, pancreatitis, hepatitis, and tendonitis are inflammation in the lungs, pancreas, liver, and around tendons, respectively.

If an area does not heal properly allowing swelling to dissipate, it can become chronic and lead to a multitude of other problems. Constant heat and swelling can damage tissues and organs. For example, inflamed tissue loses its ability to absorb nutrients, exchange oxygen and carbon dioxide, and remove waste products. This can lead to issues like irritable bowel syndrome, colitis, "leaky gut" diseases, and even metabolic disorders like obesity, insulin resistance, and diabetes. Weakened tissues are vulnerable to viral, bacterial, and fungal infections and promote cancer metastasis. Chronic inflammation will severely impair organ function and can result in diseases such as asthma or colitis.

Long-term inflammation can cause the body to harden tissues surrounding the inflamed areas in a protective effort to wall them off. This plaque buildup can cause diseases like "hardening of the arteries," Alzheimer's disease, or osteoarthritis. Long-term inflammation can even play a role in depression.

When first faced with chronic inflammation in my practice, I started to develop treatment plans that involved all the anti-inflammatory tools at my disposal—massage therapy, energy therapy, visualization, hydrotherapy (alternating hot and cold therapy), and lymphatic support. I used cooling herbs; warming herbs; herbs to improve circulation of the blood, gut, and lymph; diuretics; astringents; and mucilaginous herbs. I carefully formulated them, alternated them, and applied them topically as well as internally. All of these helped manage chronic inflammation. When I incorporated weed into the therapy plans, results improved so dramatically that I was shocked. Instead of merely managing chronic inflammation, we were curing it. For inflammation, nothing holds a candle to cannabis!

Later in my practice, I started seeing a lot of clients with autoimmune diseases. I soon realized that autoimmune conditions are connected by one biochemical condition—you guessed it—chronic systemic inflammation. In these cases, inflammation is so chronic that the body no longer recognizes the inflamed areas as part of itself. Instead, it begins to view the affected areas as invaders. Then the immune system attacks these areas and creates a vicious cycle that continues to inflame and destroy tissues.

Autoimmune diseases like celiac disease, diabetes mellitus type 1, Graves' disease, inflammatory bowel disease, multiple sclerosis, psoriasis, rheumatoid arthritis, systemic lupus, and Crohn's disease are all related to chronic inflammation, and many can be mitigated and even cured with holistic cannabis therapy. Pot can not only reduce inflammation but also heal the resultant oxidative damage and rebalance the ECS. The antioxidant and anti-inflammatory superpowers of cannabis are part of her ability to protect tissue and organ function.

The patent further describes cannabis as an antiepileptic (see Charlotte's Story below for more on her antiepileptic power). Cannabis calms neuronal excitement by inhibiting the release of excitatory neurotransmitters like glutamate and increasing the release of calming neurotransmitters like gamma-aminobutyric acid (GABA). Many components of this herb, including cannabinoids THC, THCA, CBD, CBDA, CBDV, THCV, CBC, and the terpene linalool are anticonvulsant. (See chapter 3 or the appendix for more on individual cannabinoid functions.)

Charlotte's Story

Twins Charlotte and Chase Figi were born October 18, 2006, in Colorado. At the age of three months, Charlotte had a seizure that lasted about thirty minutes. A barrage of tests found nothing. A week later, she had a second, longer lasting seizure. Then another and another lasting from two to four hours each. Although she was put on seven different pharmaceutical drugs including addictive barbiturates and benzodiazepines, the seizures got worse. So did the side effects for the toxic medications. She was in and out of the hospital and was eventually diagnosed with Dravet syndrome, or myoclonic epilepsy.

By age two, Charlotte started declining cognitively as well—a result of the medications as well as the disease. By three, she lost the ability to walk, talk, and eat and was having three hundred grand mal seizures a week. Her heart had stopped a number of times. Her mother, Paige, would give her CPR until an ambulance arrived. Charlotte was five when they signed a do-not-resuscitate order and said their goodbyes.

Then Charlotte's father Matt found a video online of a California boy with Dravet syndrome who was being successfully treated with cannabis. They fought their way through a system that was still demonizing cannabis—especially for children—and obtained a high-CBD/low-THC cannabis concentrate. The first time Charlotte tried the medicine, she didn't have another seizure for seven days! Can you imagine how her parents felt?

Charlotte then received four milligrams per pound of body weight twice daily and her seizures were reduced from 1,200 a month to two or three per month. She began walking, talking, riding her bike, and feeding herself.

"I literally see Charlotte's brain making connections that haven't been made in years," Matt said. The marijuana strain that saved her? It's now called Charlotte's Web.

"[Before cannabis] I didn't hear her laugh for six months," Paige said. "I didn't hear her voice at all, just her crying." Matt added, "[After cannabis therapy] I want to scream it from the rooftops. I want other people, other parents, to know that this is a viable option."[5]

Sadly, Charlotte died in April 2020 from COVID.

Marijuana medicine has many additional healing properties not mentioned in the patent. (As an example, see the section on cancer in chapter 5.) One important property is pain relief. There are many types of pain, including inflammatory pain, muscle-spasm pain, microglial pain, neuropathy, and, although science has yet to pin down the process, emotional and spiritual pain as well.

Pain is a complex multistep chemical pathway modulated by the ECS. It starts with damaged cells releasing excitatory, pain-signaling neurotransmitters like substance P and glutamate, which travel to the brain. Cannabis and endocannabinoids bind to vanilloid (TRPV1) receptors to inhibit the release of pain signals. Cannabis also modulates our pain-blocking opioid receptors, boosting the power of our endorphins or synthetic opioid medications.[6] This is why people can often reduce their dosages of opioids or quit using them altogether when cannabis is added to their therapy.

When injury occurs, the body produces endocannabinoids and receptors nearby. They in turn stimulate the production of endorphins and more endocannabinoids. When cannabinoids, specifically 2AG, anandamide, THC, and caryophyllene, bind to CB2 receptors, they slow the release of inflammatory cytokines and reduce pain due to inflammation. They also protect neurons from oxidative damage, preventing microglial pain and neuropathy. These are just a few examples of the different biochemical pain pathways that cannabis can inhibit. There are many more ephemeral routes that cannabis uses to help us withstand emotional pain, making her the best holistic pain remedy available.

As we have seen, within an animal's body, the ECS establishes and maintains homeostasis (balance), which enables all body systems to function optimally and is necessary for health. Most illnesses and ailments stem from an instability or weakness in the ECS. This led Dr. Ethan Russo* to coin the term *endocannabinoid deficiency syndrome* in 2008.[7]

People heal and revitalize by supplementing their ECS with marijuana, but how does the ECS system become deficient in the first place? Partially because we live in such a toxic environment and partially because people do not take good care of themselves.

MAINTAINING A HEALTHY ECS

In my practice the advice I offer for maintaining full function of one's ECS is to adopt good, basic, holistic, healthy habits: avoid toxins, exercise daily, get enough rest and sleep, and eat right.

---

*Dr. Russo is a board-certified neurologist, psychopharmacology researcher, and former Senior Medical Advisor to GW Pharmaceuticals. He is past president of the International Cannabinoid Research Society and former chairperson of the International Association for Cannabinoid Medicines. He has extensively studied the historical and cultural uses of cannabis therapy for women and summarized them in a paper, "Cannabis Treatments in Obstetrics and Gynecology: A Historical Review." He believes that cannabis extracts may represent an efficacious and safe treatment for a wide range of conditions in women that interfere with fertility, a healthy pregnancy, and childbirth.

What to Eat

Eat well. Adopt a diet rich in fresh organic produce, herbs, teas, and spices. Limit carbohydrates and alcohol. Consume only fresh, high-quality fats and oils. Consume fermented foods or other probiotic foods regularly. Drink pure water. Eliminate sugar, corn syrup, genetically modified foods, and packaged foods. Everything you consume and every bit of exercise and stress in your life affects your ECS and your health. Below are some additional dietary suggestions.

Eat weed. Consume fresh cannabis leaves or flowers whenever available. They contain cannabinoid acids in addition to protein, minerals, fiber, antioxidants, flavonoids, essential oils, and chlorophyll. They are not psychoactive because the THC has not been decarboxylated by heat or time. If it works for you, use psycho- or spirit-activing cannabis for resting your mind and relaxing your body. Use it to enhance creativity, spiritual connection, communing with nature, recreation, sleep, meditation, and general holistic health.

Eat hemp seeds and hemp oil. Hemp oil (and fish oil and other omega-3 fatty acid sources) stimulates the creation of endocannabinoids and cannabinoid receptors. Polyunsaturated fatty acids are the chemical precursors to endocannabinoids and support neurological function, retinal development, and overall health by increasing CB1 receptor gene expression. These high-quality oils also clear out toxic oils, like the trans-fatty acids found in margarines and other packaged foods. These toxins cloud nerve synapses and slow down nerve transmission, thinking, and action. There is a strong connection between deficient omega-3 fatty acid intake, poor endocannabinoid function, and mood. In short, junk food can make you dumber and sadder, while pot can make you smarter and happier!

Eat your broccoli. Studies show that diindolylmethane, found in cruciferous vegetables, activates CB2 receptors and reduces inflammation. All fresh fruits and vegetables are full of antioxidants and flavonoids that boost the ECS.

Drink herbal teas. Medicinal herbs of all kinds support ECS health. Some produce phytocannabinoids and others produce compounds that mimic cannabinoid function. Here are a few examples: Compounds in kava tea, known for its calming effect on anxiety, activate CB1 receptors. Alkyl amides, found in echinacea, have been shown to reduce inflammation by binding to the CB2 receptor and increase the effect of endocannabinoids. *Ruta graveolens,* commonly known as rue, is another medicinal herb that binds to cannabinoid receptors, and so does electric daisy (*Acmella oleracea*). Helichrysum, in the sunflower family, has anti-inflammatory, antidepressant, and antioxidant properties, and produces the phytocannabinoid cannabigerol, the precursor for all other plant cannabinoids. A liverwort plant called *Radula perrottetii* produces a cannabinoid similar to THC called perrottetinene.[8] Common black pepper (*Piper nigrum*) is cannabimimetic, although it is not as powerful.

Eat fermented foods. They contain probiotics like lactobacillus acidophilus, which increase the expression of CB2 receptors.

Eat more dark chocolate! Dark chocolate contains anandamide (which makes anandamide an endocannabinoid and a phytocannabinoid, too) and compounds that inhibit the breakdown of anandamide. It is also rich in antioxidants and low in sugar. Paired with nuts for protein, it is an ideal daily snack.

Drink alcohol moderately or not at all. It reduces the efficiency of ECS signaling.

Additional ECS Boosters

Essential oils: Stop and smell the flowers! Caryophyllene (a terpene and a cannabinoid), found in ganja and many other herbs and spices, binds to cannabinoid receptors. It has anti-inflammatory, neuroprotective, antidepressant, antianxiety, and anti-alcoholism effects, and it can also help reduce neuropathic pain through the CB2 receptor.

Cold water: Swim and take cold showers. Both improve ECS signaling.

Stress mitigation: Long periods of high cortisol levels, such as those caused by chronic stress reactions, reduce CB1 receptor expression and thus cannabinoid binding potential. Chronic psychological stress also reduces endocannabinoid levels in the brain. Breathing exercises, meditation, communing with nature, hot soaks, and listening to music can all help reduce stress, and they can all be enhanced by using marijuana.

Exercise: Medium- and high-intensity exercise activates the endo-cannabinoid system. Research also shows that exercise significantly upregulates CB1 receptors and enhances CB1 receptor sensitivity, which is one way that exercise can protect against the consequences of stress. It is also why one can get really high smoking a joint after a long hike!

Touch: Touch and touch therapies like osteopathy, massage, and chiropractic care activate the ECS.

Sleep: The ECS needs daily periods of deep rest and good quality sleep to stay healthy. Ganja helps both.

To summarize, the endocannabinoid system works on the cellular level and is responsible for keeping animals in homeostasis. It is constantly working to help us eat, relax, sleep, and forget, and to protect us from disease, illness, and oxidative damage. Cannabinoids, both endogenous and plant-produced, prevent and treat a wide range of issues including cancers and other wasting diseases, oxidation-associated diseases, chronic inflammation and associated diseases, autoimmune diseases, seizure disorders, pain, muscle spasms, eating disorders, and more (see chapter 5). When the ECS experiences weakness or deficiencies, it can lead to a broad range of issues, reflecting its broad function. Good healthy living practices, like those outlined above, and supplementation with marijuana help maintain a healthier ECS, and thus a healthier self.

2

Truth and Reconciliation

Moving beyond Propaganda and Persecution

Children of a future age,
Reading this indignant page,
Know that in a former time
Love! Sweet Love! Was thought a crime.

WILLIAM BLAKE, "A LITTLE GIRL LOST"

Despite millennia of use, the banning of cannabis in the twentieth century brought with it an explosion of misinformation and a worldwide proliferation of negative propaganda. The great war on drug users started with xenophobic politicians and soon infused the medical community. Compounding that, in the early 1970s, "back-to-the-landers," among others, began clandestine cultivation and breeding in the Emerald Triangle of Northern California. New strains proliferated on the black market, but growers were not formally tracking genetics and named their new strains unscientifically. THC was the only known chemical in their plants, so breeding was directed towards the most potent high, and cannabinoids other than THC were unknowingly bred out. Although much of this is being rectified today, the majority of the medical community is still woefully ignorant of the healing power of this herb. New medicines proliferate without regulation, and we have inherited very confusing information concerning plant strains and the classifications of indica and sativa. All of this makes our medical choices complex and downright mystifying for the new user. In this chapter I address misconceptions that have persisted from the war on drugs, discuss risks associated with contaminated medicine, and describe how to avoid or mitigate the actual side effects that can occur when using marijuana.

In the early 1840s Irish physician William O'Shaughnessy brought Indian hemp to the West as a medicine for pain and nausea. By 1850 it was added to the U.S. pharmacopoeia as a prime medicine for over one hundred separate illnesses and diseases, and cannabis medicines were being produced by pharmaceutical companies and prescribed by doctors and veterinarians. In the 1970s, it was made illegal. What happened?

THE WAR ON DRUGS

By the start of the twentieth century, racism against Latinos was already thriving in the United States. The first cannabis prohibition legislation was in Texas in 1903, and it was only applicable to Mexicans. After the Mexican Revolution of 1910, when Mexican immigrants flooded into the United States—and introduced marijuana to immigrant barrios and black neighborhoods—politicians began to take notice.[1]

Cannabis prohibition began in earnest with a government enforcer named Harry Anslinger, who in the early 1920s was in charge of enforcing alcohol Prohibition. By the late '20s Anslinger read the writing on the wall and knew the end of Prohibition was coming. He wanted to preserve his lucrative and powerful position, so he created a new threat to America's safety: weed.

In 1930, President Hoover appointed Anslinger to the helm of the newly created Federal Bureau of Narcotics. An astute judge of Washington's ways, Anslinger's campaign against pot lumped together medical cannabis, street weed, and industrial hemp. He quickly aligned himself with influential politicians and corporate bigwigs like media, timber, and papermill mogul William Randolph Hearst; nylon and plastic producer Lammot du Pont of the DuPont chemical company; and a variety of pharmaceutical corporations, all of which had a financial interest in defending their empires from hemp before she could replace their products. After all, one acre of hemp, an annual crop, could produce as much paper as four acres of mature trees and could also be made into about five thousand different products—from clothing and food to fuel and construction timber. In 1941 Henry Ford built the first car made from, and fueled by, hemp, remarking, "Why use up the forests which were centuries in the making and the mines which required ages to lay down, if we can get the equivalent of forest and mineral products in the annual growth of the hemp fields?"[2]

It was all about the propaganda, and Anslinger was a pro. Since cannabis medicines were widely popular with medical doctors at the time, Anslinger changed the name cannabis to its Mexican moniker, "marihuana." Physicians did not realize that marijuana was actually one of their favorite medicines and were not invited to participate in the process to make it illegal. Anslinger knew that the new name would also instill more fear in the white community, where he was busy connecting marijuana with violence, insanity, crime, interracial sex, and promiscuous daughters. His propaganda culminated in the 1936 movie *Reefer Madness,* now a cult classic due to its ridiculous portrayal of pot smokers.

Backed up by the U.S. government, Anslinger also used marijuana as an excuse to harass Latinos and black people, using statements like, "Reefer makes darkies think they're as good as white men," and "You smoke a joint and you're likely to kill your brother."

He also demonized music that wasn't "white," especially jazz. In 1930 Anslinger arrested jazz musician Louis Armstrong, who had talked about using cannabis to relax and make "you forget all the bad things that happen to a Negro."[3]

Newspapers, whether they believed it or not, went along for the ride, running headlines like "Murders Due to 'Killer Drug' Marihuana Sweeping the United States."[4]

Fooling most of the people all the time, Anslinger's efforts culminated in the passage of the Marijuana Tax Act in 1937, which effectively made marijuana illegal. When the legislation was presented on the floor of the House for a vote, a representative from upstate New York asked, "Mr. Speaker, what is this bill about?" The speaker replied, "I don't know. It has something to do with a thing called marijuana. I think it's a narcotic of some kind."[5] When the New York representative queried the speaker as to whether the American Medical Association supported this bill, a member of the hearing committee interrupted and replied (with a lie), that they support this bill 100 percent.

Anslinger went on to institute ridiculously stringent drug laws and mandatory prison sentences for pot and many drugs, thus giving birth to both the war on drug users and the prison industrial complex. Officially named the "war on drugs" by President Nixon in 1971, the war has cost an estimated $3.3 billion annually, and well over $1 trillion total.

In 1972 a commission appointed by Nixon to study marijuana said it should be decriminalized and regulated. Unfortunately, at that time the war on drugs was in full swing so the commission's opinion was ignored, and instead marijuana was classified as a Schedule I drug (defining it as having no medical use and a high potential for abuse). Later, Nixon's aide and Watergate coconspirator John Ehrlichman revealed Nixon's nefarious motivations in *Harper's* magazine:

> The Nixon campaign in 1968, and the Nixon White House after that, had two enemies: the antiwar left and black people . . . We knew we couldn't make it illegal to be either against the war or black, but by getting the public to associate the hippies with marijuana and blacks with heroin, and then criminalizing both heavily, we could disrupt those communities.[6]

Though the war on drugs was active during the Carter administration, former president Carter stated in 2011 that he felt the war was a travesty. "The 'total failure' of the current global drug war, Carter said, has led to an increase in the worldwide consumption of opiates by

'34.5 percent, cocaine 27 percent and cannabis 8.5 percent from 1998 to 2008.' He went on to say that in the U.S., the 'single greatest cause of prison population growth has been the war on drugs, with the number of people incarcerated for nonviolent drug offenses increasing more than twelvefold since 1980.'"[7]

President Reagan brought cops into schools to teach the DARE program (Drug Abuse Resistance Education) and the intolerant "Just Say No" campaign, which in part encouraged kids to turn their parents in to the police, and took the country back to the era of distorted propaganda and forward toward wars and for-profit prisons.

Presidents Bush, Clinton, and the second Bush made no changes. Finally, in the last days of the Obama administration, there was a move toward clemency for nonviolent offenders serving long prison terms, a move to end mandatory minimum sentences, a less aggressive stance on enforcing marijuana laws, and the abolition of prison privatization on the federal level. Obama began calling the opioid crisis a public health issue rather than a criminal issue.

Then in 2016 President Trump's attorney general officially stated, "Good people don't smoke marijuana."[8]

Like many progressive ideas, marijuana legalization suffered a setback in the Trump era. In 2020 Biden came in making promises, but by February of 2022, cannabis has not been federally decriminalized, people remain in federal prison over marijuana offenses, and the plant has not been rescheduled under the Controlled Substances Act. He has continued to let states implement marijuana reform, mostly without federal intervention, but ongoing lack of clarity from the administration has caused insane complications for the industry and kept patients from getting their medicine and consumers from accessing weed.

THE LONG LEARNING CURVE

We in this country have to make up our minds—we cannot have it both ways: we cannot be both drug-free and free.

ATTRIBUTED TO DR. LESTER GRINSPOON

When the AIDS epidemic hit Northern California, the long "relearning curve" of medical marijuana began. Still underground, patients and caregivers were quick to pick up on the near miraculous benefits of smoking and brownies for HIV sufferers. Cancer patients soon caught on. Courageous activists took to the courts, the streets, and media, claiming the right to choose and use their own medicine. When California pioneered the legalization of medical marijuana in 1996, the floodgates opened, both for research and for people to come forth and tell their stories, replacing the propaganda with accurate information. The Rick Simpson Story (detailed in chapter 6) began to circulate in the late 1990s, teaching us that not only was cannabis great for the symptoms of cancer and cancer treatments, it could also cure cancer. The California Cannabis Research Medical group was established and quickly formed the Society of Cannabis Clinicians, who gave birth to the first clinical cannabis journal, *O'Shaughnessy's*. *O'Shaughnessy's* covered international cannabis research (still illegal in the United States), patient stories, and statistics gathered by a new class of physicians, affectionately known as "pot docs." Healers, growers, and medicine makers in the Emerald Triangle began our own experimentation and studies and spread the word, too.

> *Marijuana prohibition has done far more harm to far more people than marijuana ever could.*
>
> DR. SANJAY GUPTA,
> CHIEF MEDICAL REPORTER, *CNN*

COMMON MISCONCEPTIONS

There are many confusing misconceptions concerning marijuana that can stand in the way of someone choosing this magical medicine. Below I've addressed the most common ones I have run into as a healer and teacher.

The single most frequently asked question from people investigating cannabis therapy is "I have this condition, which strain should I use?"

This question is based on the misconception that strain names are consistent and accurate, and that one kind of medicine is right for everyone with a specific condition. Due to cultivation and breeding being a long-time underground venture, strain names have been applied willy-nilly according to the whims of the breeders. At this point in time, for example, a lab can receive multiple samples called Skunk, and each sample will contain completely different chemical profiles. Not to mention that each individual plant has a different holistic profile depending on everything from her ancestors (genetics) to her grower and habitat. With research, I imagine that strain names will eventually reflect specific cannabinoid and terpene profiles, but we are not there yet and that will never be the whole story.

Another frequently asked question that stems from misconceptions is "Should I use indica or sativa?"

Indicas and sativas differ due to their ancestral lines—not according to their chemical profiles or even their medicinal effects. Indicas' ancestors come from places with very short growing seasons, like the Mongolian plains or the Hindu Kush mountains, for example. They have evolved to mature quickly as small plants with wide leaves to soak up optimal amounts of sun in a short growing season. Many have developed terpene profiles with sedative and muscle relaxing properties that lead to their reputations of being relaxing, sleep inducing, and focused on the body, but that is not always the case. They are popularly used for meditation, hunting, sleep, and hospital stays.

Sativas' ancestors evolved in equatorial areas with an unlimited summer season and sunshine. They grow slowly, are tall, and have narrow leaves. Their essential oil profiles often include more uplifting terpenes and oils that sharpen mental acuity and memory. They have a reputation for active energy and euphoria of the mind and emotions. They are often recommended to treat depression of mind or energy. They are popular to use for exercise, connecting with nature, working, and depression.

By now, however, most commonly found pot plants are unknown crosses of the two heritages. It is rare to find a pure indica or pure sativa strain, so these attempts at classification cannot be relied on to predict their effects. Over the last four decades, dope has been bred and interbred by commercial growers who were typically breeding for high THC content and no other characteristic, so most have a high THC and low every-other-cannabinoid profile. A plant's characteristic effects are also influenced by where, how, and by whom they are grown. And finally, each pairing of an individual plant's energy and an individual animal's energy will create unique healing effects.

Because strain names and types are not dependable descriptions of a plant, the cannabis industry uses lab testing to determine cannabinoid and terpene profiles. This information is still not yet ultrareliable, as samples from the same plant sent to different labs can produce different results. Labs are not yet testing for additional medicinal chemicals like phenols, alkaloids, or flavonoids.

So my answer to both the above questions is that when it comes to choosing "strains" or plants for treatment, it is best to rely on a wide variety of organic whole plant medicine. Just as we eat a diverse diet to ensure we are receiving a full spectrum of nutrients, the whole plant medicine philosophy tells us to use as many different strains of herbs as possible to receive the full palate of medicinal components available.

Another common misconception is that marijuana is a "silver bullet" remedy and can cure a plethora of conditions all by herself. This is sometimes true, but usually untrue. I have seen cancers cured and a case of Alzheimer's reversed with nothing but cannabis juice, and diabetes and rheumatoid arthritis held completely at bay with nothing but cannabis concentrate. However, these cases are rare. As herbalists the world over will tell you, herbs work better together and as part of a holistic treatment plan that considers many herbs, diet, exercise, meditation, yoga, and so on. This means that in addition to ganja, we want to include as many other medicinal herbs in our treatment plans as we can. Because people often just want to be given a medicine, take a specific dosage daily, and be cured, doctors often comply by prescribing a synthetic cannabinoid like Marinol. Unfortunately, both patients and doctors are usually sorely disappointed by the outcome. What the doctors and scientists don't yet realize is that because these plants have evolved with us for tens of thousands of years, they have intelligently learned to produce a complex formula of constituents with incredible healing power. They know far more about healing than we do, so it is safe to trust that they are providing us with help that we do not even know about!

The biggest misconception about weed as medicine is still propagated by the U.S. government. As we discussed in the chapter on the ECS, the U.S. government claimed in its patent application that weed is medicine. Nevertheless, it stubbornly classifies marijuana as a Schedule I drug, officially defining it as dangerous, addictive, and having no medical value. They offer no evidence to back this claim, and there is ample proof to the contrary. The National Institute of Drug Abuse (NIDA) was founded in 1974 and has an annual budget of over a billion dollars, much of which has been spent on studies to prove the dangers of cannabis. Yet it has failed to provide any scientific basis for prohibition and has ignored and even suppressed all evidence of pot's benefits.

It has gradually become clear to many in the medical field that the politicized and emotionally charged atmosphere surrounding marijuana research in the United States has created a flawed, predetermined stance on the part of those funding the research—the U.S. government.

Psychiatrist Dr. Lester Grinspoon has experienced this firsthand:

Let me give you a little anecdote. Years ago, I got a call from the editor of a journal called *Depression* who asked me to give my feedback on an article on cannabis being useful in treating depression. I explored it and it seemed to be true. By the time the article was published, I noticed a new paragraph at the end that said we want the readers to know that while the studies say that marijuana is useful in treating depression, we in no way support its use for depression or any other purpose. And I said, "Why in the world did you add this last paragraph?" The editor almost started crying. She said, "Dr. Grinspoon, our lab is supported by NIDA [National Institute on Drug Abuse] and if we don't include that we jeopardize our funding."[9]

Grinspoon became aware of the effect that government control of information about weed had had on his own perceptions:

> I realized how little my training in science and medicine had protected me against this misinformation. I had become not just a victim of a disinformation campaign, but because I was a physician, one of its agents as well . . . I was fascinated by my growing understanding of how little I actually knew about this drug, and even more so by the many false beliefs I had held with such conviction. It soon dawned on me that I, like most other Americans, had been brainwashed, that I was a part of this madness of the crowd.[10]

Dr. Sanjay Gupta speaks to the same issue in his article "Why I Changed My Mind on Weed":

> I didn't review papers from smaller labs in other countries doing some remarkable research. I was too dismissive of the loud chorus of legitimate patients whose symptoms improved on cannabis. Instead, I lumped them with the high-visibility malingerers, just looking to get high. I mistakenly believed the Drug Enforcement Agency listed marijuana as a Schedule I substance because of sound scientific proof. They didn't have the science to support that claim. . . . and I now know that it doesn't have a high potential for abuse, and there are very legitimate medical applications. We have been terribly and systematically misled for nearly 70 years in the United States, and I apologize for my own role in that.[11]*

Many additional fears and misconceptions have come from U.S. government propaganda and their war on psychoactive and spiritually activating drugs. Let's address some of the "pot is dangerous" myths.

---

*Dr. Gupta wrote this article prior to his CNN documentary special titled *Weed*, which can be found on YouTube.

"Is weed safe for pregnancy?" is a question I regularly hear, and the answer is a resounding "YES!" There is no rationale for keeping the benefits of marijuana from pregnant women. All humans of all ages, as well as all animals, have an endocannabinoid system that is designed to merge with marijuana for the health and well-being of the organism as a whole. The question about use during pregnancy is so common and so important that I address it in depth in chapter 5.

"I can't give my child pot—their brain is still developing!" is another thing I frequently hear. Does cannabis affect a developing mind? Of course it does. Every new experience affects a developing brain and causes the myelination of new neural pathways. This includes video games, junk food, abuse, education, spiritual connection, environmental toxins, and physical activity. Cannabis can have positive effects on a developing mind by regulating hormones and neurotransmitters, protecting nerves and brain tissue, and preventing inflammation in the brain. In Jamaica, when mothers give their children cannabis tea before school, the children are calmer, better able to focus, and get better grades. (I go into this in detail in chapter 5.)

Parents and doctors have found improvement with the use of cannabis in children with brain disorders such as autism, stuttering, attention deficit and attention deficit hyperactivity disorders, and many other issues of the mind. There are also documented cases of cannabis curing brain tumors in children. (See chapter 5, in the discussion of cancer.) International research has also shown promising results in children with Tourette syndrome. German physician Kristen Müeller-Vahl, M.D., speculates that "the positive effect in children with Tourette syndrome may be even stronger [than in adults]." She has seen the condition of an eight-year-old patient improve greatly, which she attributes to the "possibility of the developing brain being altered before the symptoms of Tourette syndrome have taken full effect."[12]

Jaime's Story

Jaime was fifteen when he first came to see me. He had suffered from a severe stutter since he was quite young and had been in speech therapy since he was ten. We talked for a long time about how his stutter affected his social life at school.

"I am happiest when I am playing soccer. On the field we don't talk, and I am not slowed down by my talking. I never talk in class, and the teachers don't call on me. I like my speech therapist, but things have not gotten better. I do like a girl in my class, but I am afraid to talk to her."

I asked him if he had ever smoked pot. He said yes, at a party once with friends. I asked if it helped his stutter, and he shyly said yes. With more discussion it became clear that the pot had seemed to slow his thoughts and focus his attention on one thought at a time. "Words just flowed out easier. I only talked better to one person; I was still scared to talk in a group."

Jaime did not feel that his family would support him smoking, so he considered other options and decided to try a tincture and started with one made from raw weed that contained mostly tetrahydrocannabinolic acid (THCA), which is non-psychoactive. There was not much effect, if any, even when he increased the initial dose. Then he tried a low dose of CBD-rich tincture, which provided more of a calming effect to his thoughts, but his stutter stubbornly clung to his tongue. Again, increasing the dose did not seem to help. Since we knew that smoking THC had helped the most, he then tried a THC-rich tincture, and his stutter was significantly reduced. He continued to experiment over time and discovered that edibles provided a less immediate but much longer lasting effect. For the next two years of high school, he used a combination of THC-rich tincture, edibles, and smoking at social events. His stutter disappeared when he had THC in his system, and his schoolwork improved immensely. By the end of his senior year, he had "outgrown" the stutter completely and was no longer seeing the speech therapist. He now works full time for a landscaping company and will soon marry that girl that he liked.

Beyond pot's effects on a developing mind, let's ask, "How does marijuana affect developing spirits?" I cannot count how many adults in my practice have shared with me that without marijuana, they would not have made it through their teenage years. She helped these teens with social anxiety, anorexia, endometriosis, abusive situations at home, and decisions about pregnancy. She helped some to develop their creativity in music, writing, theater, or the arts. She helped them find self-knowledge in the maelstrom of social pressure, parental judgments, bullying, new schools, and addiction. They became stronger in who they were as individuals, a process that I call "boosting their spiritual immune system." They were lucky to have had access to Mary Jane when they needed her, but it is never too late to boost your spirit! (See chapters 4 and 10 for more on how ganja is used spiritually.)

Another common and uninformed judgment among nonusers is that pot and parenting shouldn't mix. For many parents, the opposite has proven to be true.

According to cannabis clinician Marian Fry, M.D., writing in a 2007 survey in *O'Shaughnessy's: The Journal of Cannabis in Clinical Practice*, pot-smoking patients with parenting problems saw an "enhanced flexibility and an ability to identify the child's needs as those of a separate and unique individual . . . The parent becomes present and the child benefits from the increased positive attention. . . . Patients say cannabis makes them less self-centered and egocentric and more aware of the needs of other people."[13] Or, as many happy Emerald Triangle parents claim, anyone who says it's bad to be a stoner parent has either never been a stoner or never been a parent!

Despite many attempts by politically motivated research to prove otherwise, there exists no evidence of chronically impaired neuropsychology due to pot. Although smoking ganja has a bad reputation for harming the memory, it turns out that memory under the influence of marijuana is actually more intense due to a greater flow of oxygen and circulation to the brain. (In chapter 4 we look at examples of pot improving cognitive function in dementia patients.)

Often deeper-lying or hidden memories are brought to the surface coupled with a new, wider perspective and greater consciousness. However, because THC marijuana invites one to focus on one thing at a time, multitasking skills do tend to fall away under the influence.

Smoking herb also has a reputation for stealing motivation and productivity. The latest science claims that 5–6 percent of the population has "amotivational" syndrome, but there is no significant connection with cannabis use.[14] Consider that our society overvalues production and workaholism. Not all people believe in the Puritan work ethic, and no one should be judged against those values. There are surely lazy potheads, but there are also many ambitious and productive potheads as well as many lazy nonusers. A list of motivated, successful, and influential people thought to have smoked pot includes Barack Obama, Oprah Winfrey, Carl Sagan, Bill Clinton, Clarence Thomas, Stephen Colbert, Jon Stewart, Jay-Z, John Kerry, George Soros, Bill Maher, Bill Gates, and George W. Bush. In India, laborers take ganja breaks to energize them for more work. There is plenty of evidence, including thousands of years of human experience, to show that pot can make you creative, active, and influential rather than apathetic. An estimated 76 million Americans have used cannabis, and more than 10 million of us use it regularly. If we all lacked motivation, the country would likely come to a screeching halt. To quote my friend Doug, a contractor and community thespian, "Sure, pot makes me lose motivation—motivation to do things that suck."

Another misconception about pot is that she is addictive. This depends on the very controversial definition of addictive. First, substances are not addictive, but some people get addicted to substances. Many people can use drugs like heroin, cocaine, tobacco, and methamphetamine occasionally and never get addicted. I try not to confuse "addictive" with the ability to build up a tolerance to a substance. So, although people definitely build up a tolerance to opioids or alcohol, that doesn't make these substances addictive for all users. Although tolerance can be built up to some effects of marijuana, she is not an addictive substance and people prone to addiction rarely choose cannabis as their only drug.

Unfortunately, mainstream psychiatric medicine still believes that ganja is addictive and bad for mental health. It has even coined a name for it: cannabis use disorder (CUD). CUD is in the *Diagnostic and Statistical Manual of Mental Disorders* (DSM, published by the American Psychiatric Association) and in the *International Classification of Diseases* (ICD, published by the World Health Organization). These tomes are relied upon by clinicians, researchers, psychiatric drug regulation agencies, health insurance companies, pharmaceutical companies, the legal system, and policy makers. The DSM evolved from psychiatric hospital statistics and from a United States Army manual.[15]

Critics of the DSM and the CUD definition, among them the National Institute of Mental Health, argue that the DSM represents an unscientific and subjective system. They disavow the validity and reliability of the psychiatric diagnostic categories, such as CUD, the reliance on superficial symptoms, the use of artificial dividing lines between categories and from "normality," cultural bias, and "medicalization of human distress." The publication of the DSM now makes the APA over $5 million a year, historically totaling over $100 million. Let's take a critical look at their cannabis "disorder."

The DSM defines CUD as "the continued use of cannabis despite clinically significant distress or impairment." It does not further define distress or impairment, nor does it provide any examples. It also states: "It typically includes a strong desire to take the drug, difficulties in controlling its use, persisting in its use despite harmful consequences, a higher priority given to drug use than to other activities and obligations, increased tolerance, and sometimes a physical withdrawal state."

This is a general description of addiction and is difficult to apply to habitual ganja users. If cannabis makes folks feel better (i.e., healthier and happier), they are going to have a strong desire to use it. What are the "consequences" that are considered harmful? There is no evidence that an increased tolerance to THC causes harm; in fact, sometimes it benefits a user to increase their tolerance so that they can increase their therapeutic dose. Physical withdrawal symptoms are always short-term and minor, when they exist at all, and usually consist of altered sleep patterns or digestion. When you suddenly deprive the endocannabinoid system of long-term phytocannabinoid supplementation, it will take it a few days to adjust. The DSM reflects many of the negative myths that have been perpetuated about pot, claiming that she causes "significant impairment in academic or occupational functioning." There are hundreds of thousands of high-functioning students, teachers, and professionals that are habitual users. Pot also helps many users understand and face the fact that their school or job may not be right for them. As far as causing "some to develop suspiciousness, or social withdrawal," weed can augment what is already there, but it does not cause these symptoms. (See "Anxiety-Based Conditions" on pg. 90 in chapter 4.)

The claim that ganja use impairs driving may be true for inexperienced users, but it is not true for many habitual users. To claim that it causes "impulsivity, dangerous risk taking, and irresponsibility" without providing evidence is simply irresponsible. Many of these allegations are problems only in the eye of the beholder: impulsivity is not a disorder; dangerous risk taking is not a side effect of marijuana use; and one person's irresponsibility might be another's "seeing through society's unhealthy bullshit." To reinforce propaganda that claims "marital and/or child neglect, legal problems, impaired judgment, decreased short term memory, impaired learning, and apathy" is ignorant. Ganja use does not cause marital/child neglect; in fact, it often improves relationships. And as I've already stressed, there is no evidence that cannabis use has a long-term effect on memory, impairs learning, or causes apathy. To the DSM's assertion that "cannabis can cause disturbance in attention and awareness" (i.e., reduced ability to direct focus, sustain, and shift attention and reduced orientation to the environment), I would counter that turning one's attention inward is not a disorder. (See "Attention Deficit Hyperactivity Disorder" in chapter 4.)

What particularly alarms the psychiatric professions are the DSM's claims that cannabis intoxication can cause psychosis, including delusions and hallucinations, and triggers schizophrenia in 4 percent of regular users. Cannabis is not a hallucinogen and does not trigger schizophrenia in those who don't already have it. (See "Schizophrenia and Psychosis" in chapter 4.) To quote ethnobotanist Terence McKenna, "Drugs induce paranoia and psychosis in people who have never taken any."*

The DSM's true claims, that pot causes "disturbance in perception, relaxation, sleepiness and mild euphoria," are examples of excellent tools for mental health rather than cause for alarm.

That said, I have recently run into a group of people that have cannabinoid hyperemesis syndrome (discussed later in this chapter). These patients struggle to stop using cannabis even though it makes them extremely ill. In my definition, this makes them addicts, but does not make pot an "addictive substance."

Doesn't pot kill brain cells? No. This is another unsubstantiated rumor spread by the war on drugs. Indeed, consider the fact that the Israeli army equips soldiers with cannabis in case of sarin gas attack. That is because, contrary to the propaganda, weed is a neuroprotectant that shields the brain and nervous system from toxic and traumatic attacks.[16] Research on cannabis users is quite rare, but that done with heavy pot users in Jamaica and Costa Rica found no evidence of abnormalities in their brain physiology. Dr. Grinspoon, who has studied cannabis for more than forty-five years, has said of the old "pot kills brain cells" myth: "I've found no data for this contention. A lot of cognitive studies were compromised. Marijuana is a thought generator. The mind is always shooting out thoughts, but with marijuana they shoot out in greater frequency. It shoots out many bad ideas and many good ideas. But it generates ideas."[17]

Cannabis use can actually contribute to problem-solving in significant ways. It can help you to see your way around some corners that you haven't been able to navigate before.

---

*Terence McKenna was an ethnobotanist, mystic, psychonaut, lecturer, author, and advocate for the use of psychedelic drugs. His books include *Food of the Gods: The Search for the Original Tree of Knowledge—A Radical History of Plants, Drugs, and Human Evolution; The Evolutionary Mind: Conversations on Science, Imagination & Spirit; The Invisible Landscape: Mind, Hallucinogens and the I Ching;* and many other books and writings.

There are many intelligent, contributive, and influential people in society who smoke marijuana and who not only show no signs of brain dysfunction but excel fully in their fields. To quote visionary businessperson and philanthropist Peter Lewis: "Running a business turns out to be a pretty lonely thing to do. Marijuana would help me commune with myself. It would turn my daily collection of information into some kind of understanding of what was really going on—what the key components were, what the emotional components were. It made me better at my job . . . it basically helped me be better at almost anything I ever did."[18]*

Carl Sagan, for another example, used marijuana as an idea generator and to better understand himself and society. He wrote:

> Existential perception of the absurd comes over me and I see with awful certainty the hypocrisies and posturing of myself and my fellow men . . . Cannabis brings us an awareness that we spend a lifetime being trained to overlook and forget and put out of our minds . . . I am convinced that there are genuine and valid levels of perception available with cannabis (and probably with other drugs) which are, through the defects of our society and our educational system, unavailable to us without such drugs. Such a remark applies not only to self-awareness and to intellectual pursuits, but also to perceptions of real people, a vastly enhanced sensitivity to facial expression, intonations, and choice of words which sometimes yields a rapport so close it's as if two people are reading each other's minds.
>
> The cosmos is within us. We are starstuff. We are a way for the universe to know itself.[19]

"You shouldn't mix pot with your meds" is another misconception. One should always inform their prescribing physician when using cannabis therapy, especially in cases of very high dosage of CBD. High amounts

---

*Peter Lewis was a major donor to the Guggenheim Museum and Princeton University and Case Western Reserve University. He supported the ACLU and the Marijuana Policy Project. He died in 2013.

of CBD often increase the efficacy of pharmaceuticals, including opioids, allowing patients to reduce their dosages of prescription drugs. Specifically, CBD can deactivate certain liver enzymes, thereby altering metabolism of painkillers, statins, blood thinners, insulin, and other drugs. In these cases, patients need to be monitored to prevent overdosing on their prescription drugs. In some cases the opposite occurs, and pharmaceutical medicines interfere with the effectiveness of marijuana medicine. In animals, for example, Tamoxifen, often prescribed for breast cancer, competes with CBD attachment to cannabinoid receptors and thus interfere with cannabis treatment. On the other hand, CBD increases the effectiveness of Tamoxifen, so it depends on how you look at things.[20]

According to Project CBD, "Patients taking Big Pharma meds should monitor changes in blood levels and, if need be, adjust dosage. Problematic interactions are more likely when consuming high doses of CBD isolate products [versus whole plant medicine]."*

In general, most cannabis clinicians agree with Dr. Franjo Grotenhermen, the director of the International Association of Cannabis as Medicine: "Although pharmacokinetic interactions with other medicinal drugs can occur with very high doses of THC or CBD, these are very rare cases. THC and CBD have been given to millions of patients using other drugs without serious side effects."[21]

One drug that needs caution when mixing with high-THC edibles or strong THC concentrates is alcohol. The combination can cause the same symptoms that an overdose of alcohol or THC can cause alone—namely, nausea, vomiting, the room spinning, and loss of balance. This warning is especially for new users of either drug, but I have seen many instances in which habitual pot smokers consume an edible and then become extremely drunk from one drink or have a sudden drop in blood pressure and then pass out. In general, it's best to avoid alcohol when consuming THC edibles or strong doses of THC.

---

*Project CBD is a California-based nonprofit dedicated to promoting and publicizing research into the medical uses of cannabidiol (CBD) and other components. Project CBD was conceived in 2010 by two journalists who had been covering medical marijuana in the pages of *O'Shaughnessy's: The Journal of Cannabis in Clinical Practice.*

POTENTIAL CONTAMINANTS
IN UNCLEAN PRODUCT

Organic, sun-grown herbs and the products made with them are by far the best choice for personal health and the environment. Medicine should not contain agricultural pesticides, fertilizers, metals, petroleum products, or mold or mildew. Indoor-grown plants require a huge amount of chemicals and electricity. Even light-deprived or "light-dep-grown" plants require a massive number of single-use plastic tarps to hide them from the sun. All that causes pollution when it is created, as it is used, and when it is discarded. It causes harm to all of Earth's creatures including yourself. Instead, insist on outdoor organic herb and medicine. Be aware that the industry calls whole plant medicine "full spectrum extracts," although these rarely contain roots or seeds.

CBD products in particular have become popular worldwide so fast that they are impossible to regulate. Products made from high-resin cannabis with a clear, trackable, trustworthy origin are absolutely preferable to products made from low-resin or industrial hemp. Hemp is a bio-accumulator, which means she pulls toxins like heavy metals, pesticides, and petroleum up from the soil and concentrates them in her tissues. (Hemp was used for bioremediation after the Chernobyl disaster.) If the hemp used in your medicine is low-resin, industrial, or nonmedical grade, that means that the manufacturer has had to concentrate huge amounts of it in order to obtain a useful amount of CBD. In the process, all of the bio-accumulated toxins are concentrated, resulting in a potentially very harmful "medicine."

Very little independent, international, randomized testing is done, and when it is the results vary widely. For example, Hazekamp Herbal Consulting in the Netherlands tested CBD products from the United States, Netherlands, and Australia and found that very few samples contained the amounts of CBD stated on the label. Many also contained THC, synthetic cannabinoids like "K2" or "Spice," and heavy metals, pesticides, and other dangerous contaminants. To confuse things further, the word *hemp* is now the legal moniker for high-resin medicinal marijuana that contains less than 0.03 percent THC. Now even high-quality, well-made CBD products list hemp on the label and it is up to the consumer to determine if it is medicinal or industrial hemp.

Another potential risk comes with using vape pens (e-cigarettes). Vaporizers that use cartridges of medicine instead of plant matter are often contaminated. In January 2020, the U.S. Centers for Disease Control and Prevention website confirmed over 2,600 cases of severe acute respiratory distress related to vape pens containing illicit cartridges that had been cut with toxic chemicals like flavorings, thickening agents, and/or vitamin E oil. These additives caused inflammation and pneumonias. Most cases were treated in the hospital with steroids. Over twenty deaths were reported. (Ironically, pure cannabis vapor is anti-inflammatory in the lungs and would probably have returned proper lung function to the patients.)

All 2,600 cases came from areas where cannabis was prohibited and people were buying black market vape pen cartridges. In none of the cases were the pens purchased from a state-licensed store. Some marijuana-legal states have now banned some additives, like vitamin E oil, MCT coconut oil, and polyethylene glycol; others, like California, have not banned any yet.

There have also been reported cases of pneumoconiosis, or "cobalt lung," which is heavy metal poisoning usually found in those who grind metal for a living. These vape-pen-related cases were probably due to the metal heating coil used inside some cartridges.

For those who choose to use vape pens, the safest have no metal coils in the cartridge, no additives of any kind, and use glass (not plastic) cartridges. Some cannabis medicine manufacturing methods, like high-critical CO_2, strip the essential oils from the product. These can be safely mixed back in later in the process. Sometimes synthetic terpenes are added instead. The consumer is left to research this. The only thing that should be in a vape cartridge is cannabis.

Some methods for concentrating cannabis use toxic hydrocarbon solvents like butane, propane, or hexane, which can contaminate the final product. These will not be listed as ingredients, and the consumer has to research the processing method. Water (used to make hash), food-grade ethanol, and carbon dioxide (CO_2) are the safest solvents used in manufacturing concentrates.

Pot plants are susceptible to botrytis mold, powdery mildew, and other funguses while under cultivation. Once harvested, the dead plant can no longer fight off infection, so they can spread even after harvest during the curing process. Improperly cured pot can also pick up a composting mold like *Aspergillus,* which leads to an ammonia-type smell.

If you buy your pot from a dispensary, it has tested clean of fungus. If not, you can usually smell if the pot is moldy. Do not smoke moldy products and definitely don't use them to make a concentrate or you will be concentrating the mold too! For people sensitive to molds, or with a weakened immune system, or with a sinus or lung condition, smoke from weed infected with molds like *Aspergillus, Mucor,* and *Cryptococcus* can cause serious infections in the sinuses, lungs, or central nervous system. The rest of us can handle small amounts, undetectable by odor, but we should all avoid inhaling mold whenever possible.

Cannabinoid hyperemesis syndrome (CHS) is a newly identified phenomenon, and with very little research its etiology remains elusive. Patients experience recurrent episodes of severe abdominal pain and cyclical vomiting, sometimes up to twenty-five times a day. An episode can last from several hours to several days, and they recur in a cyclic pattern over a period of months. Many patients end up in the emergency room and are misdiagnosed. Two deaths have been attributed to associated dehydration.[22] They are the first deaths attributed to cannabis in more than eight thousand years of use.

Although often misdiagnosed as cyclical vomiting syndrome (CVS), CHS sufferers are unique in two ways. One, hot bathing (and in five cases topical application of capsaicin cream to the abdomen) relieves their pain and vomiting.[23] Some CHS patients present with skin burns due to repeated use of scalding water. Two, when they stop using marijuana all symptoms are reduced within three days to a week. Some level of symptoms can last up to a month after cessation, as it can take that long to clear all cannabis out of the body. Symptoms return if patients start using cannabis again, but not if patients stay clean of the herb.

When tracked, most CHS cases reported revolve around heavy use of THC-dominant cannabis and it is unknown what effect other cannabinoids, or well-balanced cannabis, have on the issue. Many patients claim that they only use organic weed, although this hasn't been verified. The length of time of cannabis use prior to onset varies from a couple of months to over thirty years. Age of onset also varies widely, as does the amount of cannabis used. Although I found the minimum appeared to be two joints or two blunts (cannabis mixed with tobacco) a day, cases have been reported of up to the equivalent of ten per day. In the few cases where it has been tracked, there is concurrent drug use, most often alcohol or commercial tobacco cigarettes.

The mechanism for pot's antiemetic effect is unknown, and theories for her paradoxical hyperemetic effect are too numerous to discuss here. Proposals to explain how hot showers offer relief include increased body temperature reversing chronic hypothalamic cannabinoid receptor stimulation and diversion of blood and heat to the periphery.[24]

The most promising current research, performed by Dr. Russo, is looking for genetic mutations affecting neurotransmitters, the ECS, and the cytochrome P450 complex associated with cannabinoid metabolism. He found a few of these mutations in the twenty-eight patients that participated in the study and none in the control group.[25] I hope he continues his research.

Once again, sun-grown organic weed is the safest medicine for you and the Earth. If you can't personally know and trust the source of your medicine, look for complete product labels. They should include a manufacturing date and a batch number. They should tell you that the product has tested negative for mold and pesticides. Labels should show the cannabinoid ratio of the product, the recommended dose, and the number of milligrams (mg) of each cannabinoid per dose. Knowing how many milligrams of THC a dose contains is the only way to predetermine its psychoactivity. Just as with food, labels should state that the medicine is free of corn syrup, trans fats, GMOs, artificial coloring, flavoring, and preservatives.

POTENTIAL SIDE EFFECTS

As we discuss side effects it's important to keep in mind that what is an unwanted effect for one may be a medicinal or target effect for another. All cannabis side effects, with the exception of increased consciousness and other spiritual effects, are temporary and clear when the medicine clears from the system. In general, cannabis has a drying effect on the system. Most folks experience a dry mouth, known as cottonmouth, and many experience dry and/or red eyes from any cannabis medicine. These effects can be mitigated with beverages; chewing on something bitter, candy, or cough drops; and, for the eyes, using eye drops.

Those who use marijuana habitually rarely suffer negative consequences from long-term use, aside from whose who suffer from cannabinoid hyperemesis syndrome, as discussed previously in this chapter. However, when habitual heavy users withdraw, they might experience temporary symptoms such as mild anxiety, feeling low for a few days, reduced appetite, insomnia, sweating, irritability, or restlessness. These symptoms are not experienced by everyone, they are not permanent or dangerous, and they last only a short while. They can be completely avoided by tapering off slowly instead of quitting all at once.

Side Effects from Smoking or Vaporizing

Mild side effects, including an irritated throat, bloodshot eyes, cottonmouth, and coughing, can come with smoking or vaporizing marijuana. (Be aware of the potentially serious side effects of contaminated vape cartridges, as discussed above.) Do not use butane lighters to ignite your weed because inhaling the butane is harmful and can cause a postnasal drip and irritated throat. Stick with matches or use a magnifying glass to take a "solar" hit. Sore throats and coughing can also be mitigated with mucilaginous herbs, throat lozenges, or cough drops. They can be avoided entirely by using a different ingestion method. In our "cannabis culture" we also enjoy taking "green hits" by sucking on a joint before lighting it up. This way we are inhaling the healing essential oils and enjoying the flavors and aromas of the strain without smoke or vapor.

Side Effects of THC

Both the demonization of pot and the fear of using pot revolve around her most famous molecule, THC. Now that low-THC plants and medicines are available, this isn't as much of a problem. However, there is still quite a bit of fear around using THC for the first time, or using it again after a previous overdose. Some folks fear getting stoned because they falsely believe that it will make them stupid or out of control. Many are uncomfortable being high because it makes their heart race. For others, it can bring up repressed emotions or feelings that they are not ready to face yet. All these effects and more should be considered before trying THC, or trying it again after a bad experience. As with all spirit-altering drugs, dosage, your mindset, and your setting are very important for the outcome. It is always a good idea to have a guide present to get the most out of the experience.

THC cannabis can elevate your heart rate. Feeling your heart pounding in your chest can trigger a full fight or flight response, especially if one doesn't understand what is causing it. This can lead to feelings of anxiety and paranoia (see chapter 4) for some people. Once you understand this effect, you can avoid the anxiety pathway and use the extra energy for exercise or fun, as you would with caffeine. Most frequent users build up a tolerance to this effect and it only happens a few, initial times. For others it is always part of being high. This elevated heart rate can be rectified by including CBD in one's therapy, which moderates the high of THC and calms the heart rate.

With THC, multitasking and cognitive thinking can be temporarily impaired, which can make a new user feel dumb. According to Columbia University neuroscientist Carl Hart, cannabis has different effects on the brains of new versus habitual users. In new users, there are disruptions in memory and inhibitory control, as well as slower cognition.[26]

When high, the prefrontal cortex takes a vacation from effective planning, thinking, and coordinating. However, linear thinking can be replaced by relaxation and creativity. Problem-solving abilities can also be a welcome side effect (or the main objective) of the alternative perspectives provided by marijuana. Although studies such as Hart's show that there can be clear, pronounced disruptions like these in the new user, regular users are often immune and do not have difficulties driving or working while under the influence.

As for emotional side effects, clinical psychiatrist Julie Holland* sums it up well: "For those accustomed to avoiding life's more existential dilemmas by busying themselves with activity, slipping out of time can induce some serious psychic trauma, especially if they've been avoiding who they are for a long while. . . Whatever that emotion was helping to hide comes to the surface."[27]

So, while THC is perfectly safe—and has never killed or permanently harmed anyone—new users need to approach it with care until they become accustomed to its properties that can be physically and emotionally altering. Then they will be comfortable taking advantage of its many other medicinal properties.

As you can see, a tremendous amount of false information generated by the war on drugs in the twentieth century is still in circulation today. Much of it comes from ignorant health practitioners. Doctors (and others) who recommend against cannabis treatment know little about it. Medical schools don't teach about the endocannabinoid system, nutrition, or herbal remedies. Unregulated, exponential growth in the CBD industry allows for a proliferation of contaminated products on the market. People still fear side effects that don't exist or that are easily mitigated. It is important to continue to get the word out that thousands of years of human and animal experience show that the over five hundred and fifty chemical compounds found in hemp are not only safe for consumption but are miraculously and undeniably beneficial to the mind, body, and spirit.

---

*Julie Holland, M.D., is a clinical psychiatrist specializing in psychopharmacology. She is the author of an autobiography, *Weekends at Bellevue: Nine Years on the Night Shift at the Psych ER,* and the editor of *Ecstasy: The Complete Guide—A Comprehensive Look at the Risks and Benefits of MDMA* and *The Pot Book: A Complete Guide to Cannabis.*

When It's Your First Time . . .

If you want to commune with her spiritually, make it a
    spiritual experience.
Make every time a spiritual experience.
Are you in your favorite outdoor space?
Your most comfortable, beautiful indoor space?
Have you stated your respect for the herb?
Offered her a gift?
If you feel repelled or afraid, do not continue. Save it
    for another time.

Do not . . .
Overdose.
Have any plans.
Drive.
Work with power tools.
Hesitate to take another hit when you feel like it.
Worry if you feel your heart beat stronger.

Do . . .
Keep a creative project nearby.
Release any expectations or pressures on yourself to
    engage.
Light a candle.
Light a campfire.
Take a deep breath.
Take a slower, deeper breath.
Keep your favorite toy nearby,
A bicycle, hula hoop, frisbee, paintbrush, sewing
    machine,
in case you get inspired.
Release any expectations or pressures on yourself to
    engage.
Meditate if you are a meditator.

Space out if you are not.
Release any expectations or pressures on yourself to
   engage.
Daydream.
Pray.
Chant a mantra.
Make music.
Listen to music.
Step outside.
Listen to Nature.
Go for a hike.
Ride your bicycle.
Focus on your breath.
Focus on something beautiful outside of yourself.
Focus on something beautiful inside yourself.
Eat a piece of fruit.
Go up high for a different perspective.
Focus on the dirt beneath your feet.
Drink water.
Drink herbal tea.
Ponder that your ancestors smoked herb.

Do expect . . .
Eyes to turn red.
Coughing.
A dry mouth.
A scratchy throat.
A stronger, faster heartbeat.
To not feel anything at all,
When it's your first time.

3

Whole Plant Medicine

Although it is fascinating to break the magical cannabis plant apart and study her elemental parts and chemical constituents to see how they behave individually, this is not the most beneficial way to apply marijuana medicine. Even though THC and CBD are currently the most famous and well-researched plant chemicals, they are merely players on a team that includes over 140 cannabinoids and dozens of terpenes, bioflavonoids, alkaloids, phenols, and many other medicinal components of this very complex herb.

While each team member plays an individual and complex role in healing, with different cognitive, physiological, and even spiritual effects, we must always remember that it is when provided together that they have the power to win the game. Herbalists call this power *whole plant medicine,* meaning that using the whole herb is much more synergistically powerful than using just one part. Often one plant chemical will prevent or balance out a harmful side effect from one of its teammates. Unfortunately, when physicians moved away from herbal medicine and began isolating and concentrating single chemicals found in plants, they moved away from the edict "First do no harm." Even something as simple as concentrating the pain-relieving salicylates in willow bark to produce aspirin brings with it the potential side effect of eroding the stomach lining—something that using the whole willow plant avoids because she contains a system of plant chemicals that balances out that side effect. The same thing happened with pharmaceutical opiates when they isolated and concentrated only one alkaloid, morphine, from the plant source. Pharmaceutical opiates and heroin carry a high risk of causing respiratory arrest because a teammate alkaloid in the opium poppy plant that prevents it was left behind.

Through their studies of cannabis, some scientists and doctors are coming to understand the value of whole plant medicine. They may call it by a different name, "the entourage effect," but they are "discovering" that the different chemicals within the cannabis plant work together to produce a synergistic effect much greater than that received from a single cannabinoid, or even worse—a synthetic one. They have realized that synthesizing and concentrating THC into a pill like Marinol does not work well at all, but when a patient ingests some of the whole plant, healing can occur.

Cannabis therapy requires much, much more than THC and CBD to be effective. If you are interested in the different functions of different phytocannabinoids, see the appendix, but in these pages, we will keep whole plant medicine in mind. Humans may never have a complete grasp of how much more powerful plant medicine is than pharmaceutical isolates. Or even how much more powerful a medicine formulated with multiple herbs is than one with a single herb. We must trust the plants' innate intelligence, and our five thousand years of experience using them, and simply get out of their way so that they can continue healing.

Some of the herbal actions of marijuana are listed below to show you her wide range of available uses.

Adaptogen (increases the body's resistance to stress and promotes healthy functioning)

Adjuvant (enhances the effect of a medical treatment)

Alterative (traditionally known as blood cleansers, improves the health and vitality of the body, supports the organs of elimination, aids the removal of metabolic toxins, improves nutritional uptake, and promotes the renewal of healthy tissues)

Amphoteric (normalizes and balances optimal organ functioning, bringing an excess or a depletion state back into balance)

Analeptic (exerts a restorative, invigorating action)

Analgesic (reduces pain and inflammation)

Antibacterial (effective against bacteria)

Antibilious (corrects dysfunction of the liver, especially excessive secretion of bile)

Antidepressant (relieves depression)

Antidiabetic (prevents or treats diabetes)

Antiemetic (prevents or relieves nausea or vomiting)

Antifungal (prevents or treats fungus)

Anti-infectious (prevents or treats infection)

Anti-inflammatory (reduces inflammation)

Antimicrobial (effective against microbes)

Antioxidant (inhibits free radical reactions and repairs damage caused by them)

Antirheumatic (prevents or treats inflammation of muscles and joints)

Antiseptic (effective against microbes)

Antitussive (cough suppressant)

Antiviral (effective against viruses)

Anxiolytic (relieves anxiety)

Aperitive (stimulates appetite)

Aphrodisiac (increases sexual desire)

Aromatic (contains healing aromatic compounds, especially essential oils)

Astringent (causes a local contraction and tightening of the tissues, blood vessels, and mucous membranes; used to reduce or stop bleeding, excess excretions, inflammation, and catarrh)

Blood pressure regulator

Blood sugar regulator

Bronchial (trachea/lung) relaxant

Carcinostatic (anticancer)

Cardiotonic / cardio protectant (protects and increases the health of heart muscle)

Dermatitis (skin irritation) soothing

Digestif (aids digestion)

Disinfectant (effective against pathogens)

Ecbolic (increases labor contractions)

Euphoriant (induces feelings of well-being)

Expectorant (promotes expelling mucus from lungs)

Hepatic (liver) protectant

Hypnotic (induces sleep)

Narcotic (induces drowsiness, sleep, stupor, or insensibility)

Nephritic (supports the kidneys)

Nervine (supports the health of the nerves)

Nootropic (enhances cognitive function, memory, and learning)

Nutritive (nourishes)

Parturfacient (induces labor contractions)

Relaxant (relaxes tension)

Renal (kidney) tonic and protectant

Sedative (calms)

Soporific (induces sleep)

Stimulant (increases activity of a system or organ, increases circulation)

Stomachic (supports the stomach)

Tonic (restores, refreshes, and promotes well-being)

Trophorestorative (nourishes and restores balance to the body)

Vulnerary (heals wounds)

RAW CANNABIS AND CANNABINOID ACIDS

All cannabinoids start out in the living plant as cannabinoid acids found in the crystals on a live plant. As the plant ages, more and more of the cannabinoid acids slowly fall away. The rate at which they do so is dependent on light, age, stress, and heat. When the plant is harvested, a few more of those acids will break away from their molecules and create pH-neutral cannabinoids. When someone smokes or heats pot to a certain temperature (about 250 degrees Fahrenheit), the remaining cannabinoids drop their acids immediately. The process of dropping the acid, or carboxyl group, from the cannabinoid is called *decarboxylation*. When the cannabinoid is in its acid form, it has a very different pallet of medicinal effects than when it has been decarboxylated, or "decarbed" or "activated."

The first cannabinoid formed in a young cannabis plant is cannabigerolic acid, or CBGA—I call her "Cannabi-grandma." She in turn gives birth to THCA, CBDA, and all the other cannabinoid acids. These, in turn, drop their acids and give birth to THC, CBD, and the other cannabinoids in their neutral form. In some circles it is believed that THC can break down to yet another cannabinoid, CBN or cannabinol, through oxidation. However, I've also found studies that don't support this, so the jury is still out.

The point is that cannabinoids are not stable molecules, and when they change their form, they can change their function. This is another layer of complexity within the plant, and yet another reason to use whole plant medicine. For example, THCA is non-psychoactive and anti-inflammatory, while THC is psychoactive and is not anti-inflammatory. We can use THCA in much higher doses, or consume much more raw cannabis than decarbed cannabis, because we won't get stoned. We can put lots of fresh leaves and even buds into salad dressings, salsas, pesto, juices, yogurt, granola—pretty much any fresh foods. But heating fresh leaves or buds in any way (like putting them into hot soup), might get you extremely high, because the heat will knock most of the acids off the THCA and convert it to psychoactive THC.

In addition to tetrahydrocannabinolic acid and cannabidiolic acid, many other phytocannabinoid acids, such as cannabidivarinic acid, cannabichromenic acid, cannabielsoic acid A and B, cannabicyclolic acid, and cannabinolic acid have been isolated from plant extracts, but most of the research has been on THCA and CBDA.

When my students and clients start using fresh marijuana (usually as juice), most of them experience vast improvements in their health. Aches and pains disappear, digestive issues correct themselves, and—in some cases—so do cancers and even Alzheimer's disease! Doctors and healers in Northern California and Luxembourg have witnessed many cases of fresh or raw cannabis curing many different types of cancer, including pediatric brain cancer. We use fresh leaves in poultices to prevent infected wounds, and I include it in all my whole plant medicines. We also give it to our pets and livestock to heal their issues without getting them high. For more information on fresh cannabis, see the website of Cannabis International, an organization founded by Dr. William Courtney, a leading researcher of fresh cannabis.

Below are some examples of known functions of cannabinoid acids. (See the appendix for more about phytocannabinoid functions.)

Cannabidiolic acid (CBDA): antibiotic (and anti-MRSA), analgesic, anti-inflammatory, anticonvulsant, antinausea and vomiting, antiproliferative, antioxidant, antitumor, anticancer. Decarboxylation temperature: 248 degrees F.

Tetrahydrocannabinolic acid (THCA): non-psychoactive, anti-inflammatory (stronger than CBD), antiproliferative, neuroprotective, antioxidant, antispasmodic, antinausea and vomiting, appetite stimulant, antitumor, sleep aid, reduces prostate cancer. (THCA converts very slowly to psychoactive THC after the plant is harvested. It converts immediately upon application of heat.) Decarboxylation temperature: 240 degrees F.

Tetrahydrocannabivarinic acid (THCVA): analgesic, anticancer, possible anti-inflammatory, appetite suppressant.

Cannabigerolic acid (CBGA): the grandmother of all cannabinoids.

Cannabinolic acid (CBNA): anti-inflammatory.

Cannabicyclolic acid (CBLA): anti-inflammatory, antitumor.

ESSENTIAL OILS

Although aromatherapy, the study of essential oils, has been a science for decades, mainstream science is just catching on to the power of these volatile aromatic compounds. Essential oils are complex compounds made up of not only terpenes, the new favorite chemical of the cannabis industry, but also a host of other plant chemicals, including esters, aldehydes, ketones, alcohols, phenols, and oxides. Essential oils provide the aroma of the cannabis plant, and each compound that makes up a plant's essential oil has their own unique blend of healing benefits. These benefits are available through simple inhalation, smoke or vapor inhalation, topical applications, or ingestion. Essential oils are vital players on the whole-plant-medicine team, and they act synergistically with cannabinoids, with each other, and with all the other plant chemicals. It is good to include a wide variety of essential oils in a health plan, just as our ancestors did by continually smelling and nibbling these healing plants as they found them in nature.

Essential oils and their components are delicate, volatile, and easily destroyed by heat, light, and time. Therefore, they are only present in some forms of cannabis medicine. For example, in baked goods and cooked edibles, most of the essential oils have been lost to evaporation. This is why I recommend that when decarboxylating marijuana in the oven or on the stovetop, you use a pan with a lid so that the essential oils don't just float away. I also recommend placing herbal teas in a covered cup or container to steep them in order to recapture the oils that would dissipate with the steam.

One of the best ways to benefit from cannabis essential oil, however, is by simply inhaling or consuming fresh or dried cannabis. Isn't the first thing you do when you acquire that new bag of weed is open it up and take a good whiff of the wild perfume? This makes you feel good, but it also changes your physiology and prepares your body to absorb the plant's medicine by increasing the binding affinity between cannabinoids and their receptors and increasing the strength and duration of those bonds. If you like to smoke joints, try taking a few "green hits" before lighting up in order to get the most out of the medicine.

Borrowing research from aromatherapists, the cannabis industry is currently focusing on terpenes. The terpenes found in cannabis are also present in the essential oils of hundreds of other medicinal plants. Terpenes in general are antifungal, antibiotic, and antiviral. They kill respiratory pathogens and were the original public health medicine in the form of incense. Our ancestors burned medicinal plants as incense and tossed them on the floor as "strewing herbs," and as crowds walked on them, they released aromatic medicine into the air, killing bacteria, viruses, and funguses.

Commercially sold essential oils are concentrated, usually through steam distillation, and can be found in tiny bottles in health food stores and on the internet.

But be aware that most essential oils are so concentrated that they can easily burn tissue and cause other harm. They should be diluted with a carrier oil and really should only be used under the guidance of a healer trained in aromatherapy. However, simply inhaling the aroma of a plant is always safe.

TERPENES

Terpenes are small, very lightweight volatile molecules that easily lift off a plant when it is disturbed or in the natural course of the day. Plants use them to deter insects, as protection from environmental stress, and as building blocks for more complex plant chemicals such as hormones, pigments, sterols and, confusingly enough, even cannabinoids.

Like cannabinoids, terpenes are fat-soluble and act on receptors and neurotransmitters. They modulate serotonin levels in a much safer way than, say, Prozac. They enhance norepinephrine and dopamine activity, acting as natural antidepressants. These volatile scent molecules that give pot and many other plants their unique aroma and flavor also modulate the psychoactive and physiological properties of your weed. When people feel the sedative properties of a high-THC indica strain, or the uplifting properties of a sativa strain, they are experiencing the effects of the volatile oils in the plant, which will augment or counterbalance the effects of the cannabinoids.

Below are just a few examples of primary terpenes found in cannabis.

Alpha-pinene, one of the most prevalent terpenes found in nature, is one of my favorite marijuana aromas as it conjures the scent of walking on a carpet of fir, cedar, and pine needles. This perfume will slow the breakdown of acetylcholinesterase and leave you feeling alert and better able to remember the experience. Pinene dilates lungs, counters inflammation, and shifts you into deep breathing, which increases the oxygen to your brain and improves your memory. Both alpha- and beta-pinene are antiviral and specific for COVID.

Myrcene is among the most prevalent terpenes found in weed. You will also smell it in thyme, hops, lemongrass, and citrus. Like a pint of hoppy beer, it can make you sleepy, relax your muscles, and relieve you of inflammation, aches, and pains. Like some cannabinoids, myrcene is biphasic; that is, it can have an uplifting effect at a small dose and a hypnotic effect when more than 0.5 percent of it is present. Sativa strains tend to have lower amounts of myrcene, and indica strains tend to have higher amounts.

Limonene is another favorite of mine due to her mood-lifting effect and her ability to help other terpenes get through our skin and mucous membranes. She's found in citrus rinds as well as in cannabis and has the power to dissolve gallstones, relieve heartburn and gastrointestinal reflux, and destroy microbes and breast cancer cells. Ganja with limonene is a valuable ally for anxiety or depression. Limonene enhances the activity of other terpenes and is antiviral and specific to COVID.

Caryophyllene is both a terpene and a cannabinoid! It can interact with CB2 receptors and engage their anti-inflammatory and analgesic abilities. It is antiviral.[1]

Linalool, with its floral scent and spicy overtones, will calm anxiety and sedate the overly excited. It's also pain-relieving and antiepileptic. It would be interesting to know the linalool content of the strain called Charlotte's Web, a high-CBD cannabis famous for controlling epilepsy.

Terpinolene, responsible for the floral notes in Jack Herer varietals, also offers sedation. It is antioxidant and fights cancer.

Geraniol is part of that seductive, centering, and grounding perfume found in rose geraniums. It can prevent neuropathy by protecting our nerves.

Humulene gives hops their distinctive aroma and some of their anti-inflammatory effects. It can also suppress appetite and should be avoided for those who need to increase their nutrition.

Friedelin, found only in the roots of cannabis, acts as an anti-inflammatory, analgesic, antioxidant, and antipyretic. It exhibits mild to moderate estrogenic activity in rats and also protects the liver.

Pentacyclic triterpene ketones are also found only in the roots of the plant. They are diuretic, anti-inflammatory, and antibacterial. They protect the retinas of the eyes and the kidneys. They also kill cancer cells and modulate insulin secretion, glucose absorption, and vascular dysfunction due to diabetes.

For those who want to learn more about the terpenes in cannabis I'd recommend taking a class or reading a book on aromatherapy. Although the cannabis industry is now studying terpenes, it has not yet caught up to the aromatherapists in understanding the entourage effect of all the compounds in an essential oil and how they operate synergistically with each other and the rest of the plant.

FLAVONOIDS

The synergy between the cannabinoids, essential oils, and flavonoids in marijuana is graceful and magical to behold. Flavonoids make up one of the largest nutrient families known. It includes over six thousand brothers and sisters that are all antioxidant, anti-allergic, antiseptic, antidiarrheal, anticancer, and anti-inflammatory. Working with other terpenoids (molecules made up of terpene building blocks) like cannabinoids, flavonoids inhibit the prostaglandin inflammatory pathway. Combined with the anti-inflammatory actions of some terpenes, this triumvirate of chemicals provides a much more powerful anti-inflammatory effect than one coming strictly from cannabinoids, or from any other anti-inflammatory herb, for that matter.

So far, about twenty different flavonoids have been discovered in the leaves and flowers of weed, each with its own attributes. A few are unique to cannabis, like cannflavins A, B, and C. The total content of flavonoids can reach 2.5 percent of a plant's dry weight. Flavonoids inhibit the breakdown of anandamide in your system.

Vitexin and isovitexin are flavonoids that inhibit thyroid peroxidase and may prove to be good therapy for gout. Kaempferol prevents cancer and coronary disease. Also an antidepressant, kaempferol works synergistically with the essential oils and cannabinoids in pot to create marijuana's known antidepressant effect. Like cannabinoids, apigenin modulates neurotransmitter levels and is partially responsible for ganja's anxiolytic (calming) and sedative effects. Catechins, found in green tea, bind to CB1 receptors, making them both a flavonoid and a cannabinoid found outside of cannabis.

SEEDS

The essential fatty acids in cannabis are found in her seeds and the oil pressed from them. Alpha-linolenic acid (ALA) is a precursor for docosahexaenoic acid (DHA), an omega-3 essential fatty acid and the primary structural component of the human brain. About 70 percent of a baby's brain and 60 percent of an adult's brain is made up of DHA, and it is also the main ingredient of our skin, sperm, testicles, and retinas.

In hemp seeds and hemp seed oil (often called hemp oil), the ratio of ALA, an omega-3 fatty acid, and linoleic acid (LA), an omega-6 fatty acid, is 55:25—the ideal ratio for human development. Essential fatty acids keep the myelin sheath around our nerves and all of our cell membranes healthy and strong. They condition our skin and improve our eyesight and fertility.

Hemp seeds contain all twenty amino acids, including the nine essential ones that must be consumed in food. Edestin protein, unique to hemp seeds, is similar in structure to blood plasma. It strengthens the immune system and helps the body adapt to stress.

Hemp seeds improve intelligence, increase immunity, heal disease, and improve vision. They are mildly anti-inflammatory.

ALKALOIDS

Alkaloids are found only in the roots of weed. Among them are piperidine, a stimulant, a bronchodilator, and a sedative; and pyrrolidine, an anticonvulsant that is also used in pharmaceutical medicines for epilepsy and seizures. The exact mechanism of pyrrolidine's action is not known, but like a cannabinoid, it appears to slow down nerve transmission. These and other root medicines are discussed in detail below.

LEAVES

Although long maligned and traditionally thrown away, the leaves of cannabis plants hold their own value. Fresh or dried, they are perfect for many situations. They have a lower concentration of crystals than the flowers, which means a lower concentration of cannabinoids and essential oils, since these are produced in the sticky crystals. The age of the leaf is a factor in its potency. A leaf needs a month to six weeks to start producing crystals.

Leaves are usually much less expensive than flowers. In fact, they used to be considered a waste product, and medicine makers could obtain them for free! Because they can be incorporated into any of the forms of medicine—from concentrates to topicals to salad dressings—I encourage you to incorporate them into all of your medicines. They are also ideal for microdosing and are excellent consumed fresh. They can be dried, powdered, and put in capsules, or they can be incorporated into tea blends. They are a benefit for all animals: dogs, chickens, goats, and horses will gobble them down in their food. (For my finicky cats, I add them in powder form to butter or wet food.)

Peter's Story

Peter is a sixty-year-old man with severe arthritis pain in his knuckles. Because he is a researcher and writer, this pain continually inhibits his work. In the past he used aspirin, ibuprofen, and occasionally prescription opiates to gain enough relief, but he knew that there was a trade-off with respect to his overall health. He occasionally smoked flowers and enjoyed the pain relief but could not work due to the high. We made some simple changes in his diet, removing inflammatory foods like gluten (he was already dairy-free) and adding herbal anti-inflammatories like ginger and golden paste (turmeric and black pepper in a coconut oil base). We also added some dried pot leaves to his green tea. We found that a 50/50 mix of pot leaves and green tea gave him the relief he needed without the "high" he was trying to avoid. That was all he needed. He now drinks three cups of the tea a day and is able to work all day.

ROOTS

There are records of centuries of hemp root's use. The ancient Chinese used them as diuretics and to stop hemorrhaging in women after they gave birth. The Romans found them useful in treating joint stiffness and gout, and used them to soothe burn wounds. The ancient Azerbaijanis used root decoctions (a decoction is a concentrated tea) to treat wounds, toothaches, ulcers, abscesses, and fevers. If we look closely at these traditional uses, we can begin to guess at the medicinal qualities that the roots contain. Hemp roots have been discounted in medicinal circles because they are very low in cannabinoids, but a quick analysis of their other chemical constituents confirms that the ancients knew what they were doing.

In the first century, Pliny the Elder claimed in *Natural History* that the roots could relieve stiffness in the joints, gout, and related conditions. By the seventeenth century, the roots were used regularly for those conditions and for inflammation.

Certain alkaloids and terpenes, as well as choline and atropine, are found in cannabis roots but not in any other part of the plant. The alkaloids are the bronchodilator and stimulant piperidine and the anticonvulsant pyrrolidine.

Choline is a nutrient that plays an important role in maintaining healthy cell membranes. It is used to treat liver disease, including chronic hepatitis and cirrhosis. It is also used for depression, memory loss, Alzheimer's disease and dementia, Huntington's disease, chorea, Tourette syndrome, a brain disorder called *cerebellar ataxia,* certain types of seizures, and schizophrenia. Athletes use it for bodybuilding and delaying fatigue in endurance sports. Choline is taken by pregnant women to prevent neural tube defects in their babies, and it is used as a supplement in infant formulas. Other uses include preventing cancer, lowering cholesterol, and controlling asthma. Postmenopausal women are at high risk for a choline deficiency.

Atropine is used to relax the eye muscles and to increase heart rate during resuscitation, and it also has bronchodilating properties.

Friedelin is a terpene found in the roots. It is anti-inflammatory, analgesic, antioxidant, and a fever reducer. It exhibits mild to moderate estrogenic activity. The terpene epifriedelanol, weighing in at 20–23 mg/Kg, can prevent the growth of tumors. Other terpenes in the roots, called pentacyclic triterpene ketones, are diuretic, anti-inflammatory, and antibacterial. They protect the retinas of the eyes as well as the kidneys. They also kill cancer cells and modulate insulin secretion, glucose absorption, and vascular dysfunction due to diabetes.[2]

Other minor components of the roots include cannabisativine (2.5 mg/kg) and anhydrocannabisativine (0.3 mg/kg); carvone and dihydrocarvone; N-(p-hydroxy-β-phenylethyl)-p-hydroxy-trans-cinnamamide (1.6 mg/kg); and various sterols.

With so few studies examining the composition of cannabis roots and their medical potential, this part of the plant remains in the realm of herbalists. They are truly underground, underutilized, and underrated!

Michelle's Story

Michelle credits cannabis for saving her life after a devastating boating accident in which the propeller tore up her leg and eighteen inches of her tibia. She suffered through a myriad of surgeries and severe pain that was practically untouched by prescription medications. When she first tried a cannabis tincture, she was amazed at how fast the swell-

ing and intense pain subsided. Then, Michelle's leg took a turn for the worse when her metal pins started to cause pain and infection and threatened the loss of her leg. Rounds of antibiotics were repeated, and she feared she would end up in a wheelchair by the time she was forty. She was already smoking flower, eating concentrated hash oil, and using tinctures and topicals, but it wasn't until she started eating ground cannabis root in capsules that she found consistent relief. She said that within ten days of ingesting the root of the plant via one capsule every day, her circulation issues were completely gone.

WHOLE PLANT MEDICINE TABLE

PART OF PLANT	MEDICINAL COMPOUNDS	METHODS OF INGESTION— UNHEATED (Nondecarboxylated/ THCA)	METHODS OF INGESTION (Decarboxylated/ THC)	TOPICAL USES
Roots	alkaloids, choline	consume fresh, powdered, encapsulated, cooked, or infused into oil or alcohol	no THC present	infuse powdered root into oil or alcohol, use powder in poultices
Leaves	cannabinoids, flavonoids, essential oils	consume fresh, dried, encapsulated, or cold-infused into oil, alcohol, or water	smoke, vaporize, or heat-infused in oil, butter, water or food	infused in oil or alcohol, use powdered in poultices, use in salves
Flowers	cannabinoids, flavonoids, essential oils	consume fresh, dried, powdered, encapsulated, or infused in alcohol or warm water	smoke, vaporize, infused in warm or hot oil or butter, cooked into food, hot tea	use infused in oil, salves, or alcohol, use powdered in poultices
Essential Oils	essential oils	inhale, add to cold foods or teas	no THC present	dilute in carrier oil and add to baths, soaks, poultice, alcohol, or salves
Hydrosols	some essential oils and some water-soluble components	inhale, add to food, beverages, or alcohol	no THC present	apply directly to skin, add to baths, soaks, poultices, alcohol, lotions, or creams
Seeds	protein, essential fatty acids, essential amino acids	consume fresh	no THC present	N/A
Seed Oil	essential fatty acids	consume fresh, uncooked	no THC present	for skin and hair
Spirit	mental, emotional, and spiritual guidance	not necessary to ingest the plant to meet her spirit, but it helps	any, all, or none	any, all, or none

4

Weed for Mental Wellness

Official definitions of mental health are full of un-useful vocabulary like "subjective well-being," "self-actualization," and "reaching emotional and intellectual potential." Some definitions even include ideas like "productive work" and "respect for authority"—leftovers from harmful influences of controlling societies. Over the years I have compiled my own list of characteristics of a mentally and spiritually healthy person in order to help me identify treatment goals for myself and others.

Characteristics of Mental and Emotional Health

Healthy people . . .

Can accept and respect themselves without harsh criticism, judgment, or delusional self-aggrandizement, and they accept and respect others the same way.

Can care for themselves interdependently with family or community and cope with the usual stresses of life.

Can "enjoy the journeys" of life independently from reaching a certain destination.

Have the confidence or faith to embrace the unknown.

Have the ability to focus on the present without obsessing about the past or worrying about the future.

Have the ability to not "sweat the small stuff."

Have the confidence and self-respect to be unconventional without seeking to shock or disturb others.

Have the ability to resist enculturation and not let themselves be molded by unhealthy societal norms.

Have realized that accumulating material goods does not lead to happiness.

Have recognized an unselfish purpose in life.

Have at least a few deep, long-lasting relationships.

Recognize that all beings are connected and are part of a larger universal organism.

Have no desire—or can recognize and govern the desire—to control others.

Can feel gratitude, forgiveness, and compassion and do not become overwhelmed by emotions such as fear, anger, jealousy, guilt, joy, or anxiety.

Can be humble and are not self-absorbed.

Have the ability to set and reach short-term, realistic, and desired goals.

Can recognize and resist other's views of who one "should" be or how one "should" behave.

Hide nothing from themselves and have their unconscious mind well integrated with their conscious mind.

Have the ability to accept and even love their "dark side."

GETTING HIGH IS GOOD FOR YOU!

Regular users of Marijuana are usually high functioning adults and self-actualizers, and few members of society reach a more mature or more fully human state.

JOAN BELLO[1]*

Until now, we have discussed the role of cannabis therapy in treating illnesses and dis-ease, but we would be remiss if we didn't mention that getting high is good for those who are healthy and whole as well. Weed can enhance everyday experiences as well as life's special occasions. Psychiatrist Lester Grinspoon describes being high as "a magnification of pleasure in activities, and a catalyst of new ideas, insights and creativity. . . I cannot possibly convey the breadth of things it helps me to appreciate, to think about, to gain new insight into."[2]

Part of ganja's ability to enhance experiences comes from slowing and deepening the breath. Slow breathing increases oxygen levels, which in turn amplify auditory, olfactory, visual, and taste sensations. Another part of this effect comes from her ability to bring us into the present and to "forget" previous experience. An everyday peach suddenly tastes divine and feels luxurious sliding down your throat in a way that you have never noticed before. Another part of the enhancement effect comes from a change of perspective. You might see new interpretations of a familiar work of art or find yourself appreciating unfamiliar music, or silence, or sounds that you have always ignored. Part of the enhancement is coming into your body. Aches and pains disappear, exercise feels

---

*Joan Bello is the author of *How Marijuana Cures Cancer* and *The Yoga of Marijuana*. She became an ardent activist for marijuana over forty years ago when it helped cure her young son of epilepsy. She received her master's degree in Eastern Studies and Holistic Health from the Himalayan International Institute. She integrates her extensive knowledge of yoga science with her studies and experiences with marijuana therapy. Bellow was imprisoned in the early 1990s for possession of marijuana. After that experience, she became the director of a class action lawsuit against the U.S. government for its prohibition of therapeutic cannabis at a time when such action was considered treasonous. She continues to focus on the wonders of this ancient Earth medicine and teaches to this day.

better, and so do dancing, soft fabrics, and sex. Artists, poets, musicians, creatives, and tantric gurus have all said that such enhancement is the single most beneficial aspect of pot.

With this perspective, nonusers can let go of their judgments around "stoner" behavior and understand that what looks like laziness or "spacing out" is actually someone turning inward, feeling euphoria, and appreciating what's around them. You do not need to be ill to gain great value from marijuana in terms of insight, meditation, recreation, and creativity. As author Ken Kesey* is said to have observed: "To be just without being mad (and the madder you get the madder you get), to be peaceful without being stupid, to be interested without being compulsive, to be happy without being hysterical . . . smoke grass."

Now that we have a better idea of what mental health is and how ganja can enhance healthy lives, let's take a look at how cannabis therapy aids those who are not fully mentally or emotionally healthy.

A mental illness is a complicated, multilevel disease that causes mild to severe disturbances in thought and behavior that result in the inability to cope with life's ordinary demands and routines. Mental illnesses are holistic and usually have both physical and spiritual components and are related to, caused by, aggravated by, or a result of a variety of issues. These include excessive stress, hormonal or other biochemical imbalances, poor nutrition, dietary intolerances, self-repression of emotion, and/or being the victim of repression, persecution, torture, trauma, or an unstable upbringing. Causes and aggravating factors may also include genetic factors, physical disease, spiritual disconnection, birth defects, or

---

*Kenneth Elton "Ken" Kesey was an American novelist, essayist, and countercultural figure. He considered himself a link between the Beat Generation of the 1950s and the hippies of the 1960s. His notable works include *One Flew Over the Cuckoo's Nest*, a novel set in an Oregon psychiatric hospital that serves as a study of mental institutions and the human mind. *Time* magazine included the novel in its "100 Best English-language Novels from 1923 to 2005" list, and it also appeared on the BBC's The Big Read poll of the UK's two hundred "best-loved novels." In 1965, following an arrest for marijuana possession and subsequent faked suicide, Kesey was imprisoned for five months. He also published excerpts from an unfinished novel titled *Seven Prayers by Grandma Whittier*, which was an account of his grandmother's struggle with Alzheimer's disease.

a combination of all the above. There is often a component of physical or emotional isolation, like feeling alone in the world or unloved. Each person's illness has a unique set of physical, mental, and spiritual symptoms.

In my experience, causative factors are usually multiple and, like the symptoms, are unique for each case. Symptoms that seem to arise spontaneously can be the expression of long-term suppression of memories, emotions, or trauma. Some illnesses remain buried in the genes until a certain age is reached. Mental illness can develop under torture, chronic pain, prescribed psychiatric medications, drug abuse, head injuries, ischemic injury, chronic stress, in the womb, or from a thousand other reasons. It can range from acute and catastrophic, but also includes light symptoms that hardly interfere with life or relationships. Again, over the years I've compiled a list of symptoms that can help us recognize when someone needs therapy.

Signs of Mental or Spiritual Dis-ease

Persons with mental or spiritual illness may experience one or more of the following signs:

- Cognitive difficulties, including confused thinking or problems concentrating and learning
- Excessive emotions such as rage, anxiety, fear, depression, irritability, or unwarranted hostility
- Constant worrying
- Extreme disproportionate mood changes
- Complete social withdrawal
- The inability to connect with others or nature
- Dramatic changes in eating or sleeping habits
- An inability to cope with daily responsibilities, problems, and activities
- Suicidal or homicidal thoughts
- Numerous unexplainable physical ailments
- Addiction
- Abusing other beings or harming themselves
- A lack of empathy or compassion

- Extreme self-absorption
- Hyperactivity
- Persistent nightmares
- Persistent aggressiveness, hostility, or violence toward others
- Frequent temper tantrums
- Delusions of grandeur or inferiority
- A lack of self-esteem, self-respect, or self-love
- Delusions of reality: difficulty determining what exists for every-one and what exists only in their inner world
- Hallucinations

Western society does not have a great record when it comes to treating the mentally ill. Our history is full of sadistic and malicious abuse, imprisonment, drastic experimentation, and homelessness. Modern psychiatry is a step away from that, but prescription psych meds can be extremely harmful. They are often prescribed based on an assumed and imaginary (there are no actual tests) chemical imbalance in the brain. Psychiatrists will prescribe one drug after another trying to quell symptoms. Then they add additional drugs to mitigate the side effects of the initial medication. And often a third or fourth drug to mitigate the side effects of the second medication, leading to chemical cocktails that can leave the patient obese, bloated, and zombielike, with damaged organs and body systems. These therapies are sometimes given without accompanying counseling, as if the dis-ease has no mental or emotional component. Some of these drugs can be extremely addictive. I have had clients who remain addicted to drugs like benzodiazepines or Adderall for life. If they can no longer get them, they turn to street drugs like heroin or methamphetamine. Meanwhile, these chemical cocktails anesthetize the user, suppressing symptoms at best and aggravating them at worst. Patients using these drugs become less conscious and aware, further burying the cause of their dis-ease while also causing systemic physical harm. Many of these drugs carry labels warning that they lead to homicide and suicide.

It is my sincere hope that our society will turn to counseling and natural medicines for mental illness. By fostering spiritual practices, healthy expression of emotion, integration of the unconscious with the conscious, behavioral cognitive therapy, and learning to be true to oneself despite societal or family pressure, we can help people heal without causing harm. Mary Jane, as always, is waiting in the wings to help us out.

Instead of taking five or six of the prescriptions, I decided to go a natural route and smoke marijuana.

SINGER-SONGWRITER MELISSA ETHERIDGE*
ON CARING FOR HER
OWN MENTAL HEALTH

I never would have survived my experiences traveling solo throughout Africa, and beyond, without Swazi Gold, that nurturing, outlawed weed that grew in the hills and was parceled out in matchbooks in the parks. After smoking, I found I could drop my masks and check in with my true self. Sitting in a sunny spot in the hills overlooking a stream, I found my spirit soaring with the snowy egrets as they flew across the fields of maize below. Watching the village go about its business with a bird's-eye view gave me a larger perspective. High, I could stay in touch with my true nature and connect with the humanness of it all. Swazi, British, Afrikaner, Indian, American—we were all just humans doing what humans had been doing since the beginning of time. Fetching water, herding cows, walking to school, minding the children, and doing the best we could with what life gave us. I began to recognize my prejudices and judgments and somehow the dagga helped me see beyond them, forgive myself for my mistakes, and feel a closer connection to those around me. Swazi Gold guided me to spiritual health. As

---

*The Oscar- and Grammy-winning singer-songwriter Melissa Etheridge is a cofounder of Santa Cruz County-based cannabis company Etheridge Organics, a brand targeting first-time cannabis users, especially middle-aged women who are discovering the benefits of cannabis over alcohol and pharmaceutical drugs for issues such as insomnia, anxiety, and menopause symptoms. Her love affair with marijuana began in 2004, when she was undergoing chemotherapy to treat her breast cancer.

Bob Marley is said to have said, "When you smoke the herb, it reveals you to yourself. All the wickedness you do is revealed by the herb—it's your conscience and gives you an honest picture of yourself."

Later, as my practice expanded from massage therapy and herbal remedies to holistic healing, I began to work with clients with mental illnesses. With a deeper and broader perspective, I found that much of what society termed "mental" illnesses were actually caused by a spiritual disconnect. Many people have rejected the religion they were brought up in because it did not serve them, and rightly so. Unfortunately, in doing so they also sacrificed spirituality, losing the rituals, prayer, song, meditation, offerings, ceremonies, and periods of silence that are important tools for thriving in life and for surviving life's hardships. Even many who practice a religion faithfully find no help there for situations such as abuse, depression, unresolved grief, miscarriages, loved ones with addictions, and other everyday issues.

Realizing that spiritual illness responds best to spiritual treatments, I began a more intense study of the great religions and spiritual philosophies of the world. From indigenous healers I learned about communicating directly with the spirits of nature and the ancestors and about working with people on the soul level. I intensified my studies of the energetic body and the chakra system. I acquired skills like removing curses, energetic "objects," and unwanted spirits. I learned to work with past lives (or lives in other dimensions), metaphors, and diagnostic tools like "throwing the bones." I questioned my Western herbal and bodywork teachers about the spiritual bases of their practices. I began my own spiritual practice revolving around the cycles and seasons of the Earth, and I learned how to find guides and friends within the world of spirits. I read religious and spiritual texts from Hinduism, Buddhism, Taoism, Judaism, Christianity, and the Vedic religion. I searched for commonalities around guidance for being happy and fulfilled. I found that the indigenous spiritualities and great religions of the world teach us some of the same things, including that active rituals and provoking emotions like forgiveness, gratitude, grief, and connection to nature protect us from spiritual stagnation and keep us healthy.

It was at about this point that an herbal teacher presented me with a book that opened up the world of cannabis spirituality, *Green Gold the Tree of Life: Marijuana in Magic and Religion,* by Chris Bennett. Chris proved that the most common herb used as a spiritual tool around the world was hemp. That was both a surprise and very validating for me, because pot had helped me so much spiritually throughout the years, but due to her demonization, I had thought that I was the only one!

Happiness research has shown that having a more positive outlook on life profoundly improves one's health.[3] It is no fluke that one of our inner cannabinoid molecules is named Bliss. A low anandamide level can be at the root of depression, anxiety, and fear. Supplementing with THC medicine can rebalance our endocrine system, lighten our mood, and open our hearts. Mary Jane can alleviate the physical, mental, and spiritual symptoms of "mental" illness, and then help heal the causes.

Thoughts generated in the left hemisphere are verbal, analytical, logical, competitive, and dominating. These traits are overencouraged in our society to the detriment of traits generated by the right hemisphere, which are holistic, spatial, feminine, communal, nurturing, and intuitive. Using marijuana entrains our brainwaves into alpha waves and enhances both hemispheres. She brings them into balance, literally changing brain chemistry to increase consciousness. Not only does cannabis increase our awareness of our inner world, it also enhances awareness of our outer world, our intuition.

Looking at things from the community perspective, I found that collective traumas like war and genocide are literally carried in the genes of an entire population. Experiences from our environment can cross directly into a cell nucleus and change genetic expression—which then gets passed on to our progeny, and their progeny, and their progeny. This is how our individual outlook on life can affect our great-great-grandchildren. Marijuana can help us process stress and trauma as it occurs, thus preventing post-traumatic illness and dis-ease. Pot protects us from the ischemic effects (oxidative damage) brought on by emotional or psychological abuse. Perhaps the reemergence of marijuana as medicine will disrupt these patterns and heal future generations.[4]

Biologically, restricted or shallow breathing, repressed emotions, and stress can all worsen degenerative diseases via production of pro-inflammatory chemicals called cytokines. Hostility is an independent risk factor for coronary heart disease. Stress can literally break one's heart. Ongoing anxiety raises cortisol levels in the bloodstream that increase the heart rate and release coagulation factors that can block arteries. This makes revenge, blame, guilt, hostility, grudges, and the like actual pathologies, which makes learning to feel forgiveness, compassion, sympathy, self-love, and vulnerability the treatments. When we consume weed, our breathing opens up and our hearts literally swell and grow stronger. Contractions become more robust, circulation to our entire body surges, and the sentiments we feel are more "full-bodied."[5]

How does she do it? Like Dorothy peeking behind the green curtain, Mary Jane slides under old defenses, melts down the armory, and exposes the illusions buried deep underneath. She lifts the filters that obscure self-awareness—be they a parent's opinion, your superego, or society's judgments. Harmful mental rigidity and tightly held beliefs drift away with the clouds. Our egos shrink and we are left contemplating how we are all connected. Being high simultaneously unclouds our judgment and frees us from the yoke of judgment. Mary Jane reminds us to question authority and that freedom—from governments, from abuse, from drugs—is worth fighting for.

Merely being with your emotions is the beginning of true healing.

UWE BLESCHING*

---

*Uwe Blesching, Ph.D., is a medical writer, author, and speaker in the areas of cannabinoid health sciences and mind-body medicine. He is the cofounder and chief science officer at the CannaKeys website, which is dedicated to unlocking the science of the endocannabinoid system. He is the author of *Your Cannabis CBD:THC Ratio: A Guide to Precision Dosing for Health and Wellness*, *The Cannabis Health Index*, and *Breaking the Cycle of Opioid Addiction: Supplement Your Pain Management with Cannabis*.

The folks who come to me with panic attacks, self-loathing, depression, eating disorders, and addiction often do have "chemical imbalances" in their brains, but not the kind that benefit from prescription psych meds. Their ECS deficiencies may be a result of previous trauma, unresolved grief, or self-obsession. This leads to poor connection to others and/or nature, inability to form intimate relationships, and an inability to shift out of their heads and into their hearts. Without spirituality, life's mistakes and misfortunes can pile on top of us, cutting us off from loving relationships and loving ourselves. The joy in life can begin to wither. Physical ailments often appear as our body attempts to get us to pay attention to our spirit.

Mary Jane builds mental health in a myriad of ways. For example, with obsessions and compulsions, she points out our delusions of control and provides gentle support when we need self-control. With symptoms of past trauma, she will cease the cycle of nightmares, calm the hyperaroused, and climb into bed with even the most hopeless insomniac to carry them off into a deep, healing sleep. For addicts, she will act as a safe substitute for poisonous medications and lend us the courage to examine what we are trying so hard to suppress. For anxiety, she can relax both emotional and muscle tension, help us to envision conscious responses to replace unconscious reactions, cooperation in place of competition, and community in place of division. For eating disorders, she will help us face abusive pasts, laugh away our self-loathing, and renew our appetites for life. She teaches us how to maintain the inner serenity needed to ride out the storms of life, and she provides the perfect nutrition for healing the trinity of the mind, the spirit, and the body.

The hemp plant is resilient, flexible, adaptable, and extremely strong. She can help us be that way too. She can heal us mentally and spiritually by showing us how to breathe, relax, slow down, lighten up, and laugh at the world. She gives us the spiritual tools of tolerance, gratitude, awareness, kindness, being present, and forgiveness. She enlarges our capacity for compassion and consciousness, and she activates the bliss encoded within our very being.

The next section will detail various mental and spiritual dis-eases that can be successfully treated with marijuana medicine.

ANXIETY-BASED CONDITIONS

Let's look at some common psychological and spiritual conditions and how marijuana can help. I begin with an exploration of anxiety, followed by conditions that have anxiety as a component.

Anxiety

I want to begin our investigation of mental/spiritual illness by discussing anxiety because it can be a disorder by itself and also an underlying symptom of many other mental and spiritual disorders, including paranoia, bipolar disorder, obsessive-compulsive disorder, and post-traumatic stress disorder.

When working with anxiety disorders, we often need to quell symptoms before we can explore the causes. In worst-case scenarios, anxiety attacks are sporadic, seemingly unpredictable, and debilitating. Never knowing when they will come can cause fear of going out in public, of going to sleep, and of family or social gatherings. This fear, although legitimate, adds to the cycle of stress, so first we work towards conquering the fear of the anxiety reaction itself. We do this with tools that empower someone to reduce the length of a reaction if it comes up in public or when awakened in the night.

Then we work to identify triggers. These might be situational, dietary aggravators, scents or sounds that trigger memories, certain times of the day, or certain people like bosses, exes, or family members. Once someone can quell their anxiety reaction, they know that if they have an episode while out, they have the tools to handle it. This alone is tremendous relief for a major source of anxiety!

An understanding of anxiety reactions and the autonomic nervous system from which they stem provides the basis for understanding paranoia, intermittent explosive disorder (IED), bipolar disorder, PTSD, and some cases of depression. Anxiety itself is a normal, healthy reaction to the anticipation of stressful events. It keeps us alert and ready for action and can often be confused with excitement. However, when the autonomic nervous system becomes unbalanced, and the anxiety reaction becomes stuck in the "on" position, this has a negative impact on one's mental, physical, and spiritual health.

Anxiety disorders cross cultural and historical borders. In *The Anatomy of Melancholy* (1621), Robert Burton described the symptoms of anxiety attacks in socially anxious people: "Many lamentable effects this fear causeth in man, as to be red, pale, tremble, sweat; it makes sudden cold and heat come over all the body, palpitation of the heart, syncope, etc. It amazeth many men that are to speak or show themselves in public." Hippocrates also made note of it, describing social anxiety as: "He dare not come into company for fear he should be misused, disgraced, overshoot himself in gestures or speeches, or be sick; he thinks every man observeth him." Anxiety disorders are the most prevalent mental disorders in the United States and worldwide. About 35 percent of people experience an anxiety disorder in their lifetime, and I would estimate that about 50 percent of my clients have done so. Even a single event can be debilitating, and frequent, uncontrolled episodes may make the sufferer afraid to drive or even to leave home. They are also a prime component of many other mental disorders including, but not limited to, paranoia, explosive disorders, bipolar disorder, obsessive-compulsive disorder, post-traumatic stress disorder, and addiction.

It takes a chronically activated sympathetic nervous system and a tremendous amount of energy to repress emotion, trauma, and memories. Our issues live in our tissues, and old trauma lives just behind the breastbone, well protected by shallow breathing. When marijuana use deepens our breathing, some of those issues may resurface and freak us out. Because of this, marijuana therapy may be difficult for those who fear meeting their true selves or are not conscious of their defense mechanisms. For people who are not yet ready to face their traumas, cannabis therapy can be frightening because of the intensity of the clarity it brings. Education and counseling are necessary adjuncts to marijuana therapy in these situations.

My clients seldom initially know what is causing their episodes of anxiety, but something hidden is activating their sympathetic nervous system and their "fight or flight" response. As adrenal glands release adrenaline (epinephrine), the heart rate speeds up, breathing becomes shallow, digestion is inhibited, and some may experience tremors, shakiness, and/or insomnia. In extreme cases, this nervous state becomes chronic and the adrenal system is depleted, leading to exhaustion. A stress reaction is like a turbo boost in response to danger, but if there is no real danger, or if the turbo gets stuck in the "on" position, you run out of gas quickly.

Cannabis therapy fits into this picture every step of the way. The endocannabinoid system facilitates the entire nervous system—and spiritual health. Anxiety symptoms are a sign of imbalance within the nervous system. They also signify a lack of spiritual faith and support.

To understand the effects of weed on anxiety, we must look at the autonomic (or autonomous) nervous system, the ANS, which controls unconscious bodily functions such as breathing, heartbeat, and digestion. It has two parts: the sympathetic nervous system, which prepares the body for action, and the parasympathetic nervous system, which allows for digestion and rest.

Anxiety and the fight or flight response are under the direction of the sympathetic nervous system, which perks the body up by dilating the pupils, accelerating the heart rate, constricting blood vessels, and raising blood pressure to send more blood to the muscles. Accelerated breathing gets more oxygen to the brain and muscles. The digestive system shuts down and diverts that energy to the CNS and muscular system.

The parasympathetic nervous system *does the opposite*. Think: sympathetic = stimulant and parasympathetic = relaxant.

According to Sachin Patel, M.D., Ph.D., of the Vanderbilt University Medical Center, when individuals are experiencing anxiety (or stress or trauma), their concentration of endocannabinoids decreases. "There is a reduction in both the levels of production and in the responsiveness of the receptors. Stress inhibits the endocannabinoid system and is a key trigger for the development and exacerbation of a variety of psychiatric

SYMPATHETIC NERVOUS SYSTEM	PARASYMPATHETIC NERVOUS SYSTEM	STONED NERVOUS SYSTEM
Accelerates heart rate	Slows heart rate	THC slightly increases heart rate
Induces rapid, shallow breathing	Induces slow, deep breathing	Induces slow, deep breathing
Halts digestive activity	Stimulates digestive activity	Stimulates digestive activity
Constricts blood vessels	Relaxes blood vessels	Relaxes blood vessels
Raises blood pressure	Reduces blood pressure	Reduces blood pressure slightly
Tenses muscles	Relaxes muscles	Relaxes muscles
Dilates pupils	Constricts pupils	Dilates pupils
Dries out membranes	Moistens membranes	Dries out membranes

disorders. When you consume cannabis in an anxious or stressed state, you're essentially replacing the missing endocannabinoids with a plant-based version. This causes a near-immediate relief of anxiety symptoms."[6]

By themselves, anxiety disorders can be debilitating, but they are also the base for many other mental health issues such as paranoia, intermittent explosive disorder (IED), bipolar disorder, and post-traumatic stress disorder (PTSD). For these, we start with therapy for anxiety, and then dive deeper.

Paranoia

Pot has long had a reputation of bringing on paranoia. THC is considered an anxiogenic, or anxiety-generating chemical. However, upon closer investigation, we discover that this classification is not accurate.

Looking at the table comparing the sympathetic and parasympathetic systems it is clear that cannabis actually balances the autonomic nervous system and maintains it in its healthiest state. So why do some folks feel paranoid after smoking pot? Usually, it is because they are a bit paranoid already. "Pot makes you more of who you are" is a common way to explain this. It enhances whatever you are feeling at the time. Often a new user's "paranoia" comes from fear of "getting caught" by authorities, or from fear of judgment due to the propaganda and stereotypes that demonize "stoners." With a slightly increased heart rate, dilated pupils, and a dry mouth, it can feel like your body is preparing for danger—even when no real danger is apparent. If you are already unsettled in social situations or the setting that you are in when using pot, those feelings can be amplified, and pot can make you focus on perceived threats or feel vulnerable to harm. As with all psychically active drugs, "set and setting" are very important for initiation into cannabis therapy! Your surroundings and your attitude determine your journey. (See "When It's Your First Time" in chapter 2.)

Intermittent Explosive Disorder (IED)

Intermittent explosive disorder is an impulse-control disorder characterized by sudden episodes of unwarranted anger, hostility, impulsivity, and recurrent aggressive outbursts. Those with IED explode into rages despite a lack of provocation or reason. Therapy for folks with this issue begins with therapy for an anxiety disorder. Inhaling cannabis when angry immediately slows down thoughts and relaxes body tension. It helps us focus on the present. This allows for objective witnessing and emotional distance. With weed's help we can treat outbursts immediately, work toward preventing them with diet and exercise, and repair and strengthen the nervous system. By combining cannabis therapy with counseling, people often regain control of their outbursts, freeing them to work on the root causes of their issue and heal themselves and their relationships.

Bipolar Disorder

Bipolar disorder, also known as manic depression, is a mental illness that brings severe high and low moods and changes in sleep, energy, thinking, and behavior. It is a vicious cycle that starts with a manic period that overstimulates the sympathetic nervous system. That leads to exhaustion and depression. In essence it is when two opposite parts of the personality cannot exist together at the same time. The nervous system can operate either sympathetically or parasympathetically, but not both at the same time. Psychiatric drugs can suppress severe symptoms, but are also suppressing emotions and thus contributing to the cause while doing great harm to the physiological organs and systems of the body. Cannabis therapy can help with symptoms by balancing the autonomic nervous system. Combined with counseling, patients can learn to reintegrate their two poles so that they may exist together and thus return balance to the personality.

Obsessive-Compulsive Disorder (OCD)

Obsessive-compulsive disorder is a common, chronic disorder in which someone has uncontrollable, recurring thoughts (obsessions) and develops repetitive behaviors (compulsions) as a coping mechanism to distract them from their obsession. Often patients harbor intense fear around "being discovered" as abnormal. There are few valuable studies concerning OCD and cannabis.

OCD patients are often told that pharmaceutical antidepressants and antianxiety medications are the only treatment options, and SSRIs are the most commonly used. However, they have a dismal rate of success. One long-term study showed that only 20 percent (17 of 83) of subjects had experienced a remission of their OCD symptoms at a five-year follow-up; 49 percent (41 of 83) were still experiencing clinically significant OCD symptoms.[7] Although results are slightly better when paired with therapy, the pharmaceutical-only model treats the symptoms and not the person. The pharmaceuticals' harsh side effects can include suppressing emotion and worsening of mental, physical, and spiritual health.

The most valuable report I found involved eighty-seven individuals with OCD who tracked the severity of their compulsions and/or anxiety immediately before and after cannabis use for a period of thirty-one months. They reported an average of 60 percent reduction in compulsions, and a 52 percent reduction in anxiety after inhaling pot. Higher doses of CBD seemed to lead to a larger reduction in compulsions.[8]

A small number of experiments on mice report beneficial effects in OCD-like behavior from "substances that stimulate the endocannabinoid system." However, these studies do not take into account that the animals are tortured to induce obsessive marble-burying behavior, or that synthetic cannabinoids are not nearly as effective as plant medicine, so I do not find these studies valuable.[9]

Like all serious mental health conditions, OCD takes on different personas in different people. Good therapy programs are patient specific, include counseling, and take into account a person's unique rate of adaptability, living conditions, spiritual life, and so on.

Post-Traumatic Stress Disorder (PTSD)

PTSD is a common and complex disorder that exists in all societies. It occurs in people who have experienced or witnessed one or multiple traumatic events without being able to process them in a safe place or time frame in their lives. Experiencing events such as natural disasters; accidents; war; terrorist acts; gang life; ongoing or multiple acts of physical, mental, or emotional abuse; rape; assault; or being forced to commit violent or abusive acts against one's will or morals can break down the self's ability to ever feel safe in the world. PTSD is marked by triggers that can bring back memories of trauma, causing someone to feel like they are still in that situation, and to reexperience the intense mental, emotional, and physical reactions that accompanied the original event or events.

Symptoms may include flashbacks, nightmares, hyperalertness, anxiety, fear, panic attacks, insomnia, depression, headaches, exhaustion/fatigue, inability to focus, and much more. Patients often abuse drugs or alcohol to block out memories and emotions. Eating disorders are not uncommon, as patients seek some semblance of control over themselves. Uncontrolled outbursts of temper and violence and damaged intimate relationships and a sense of isolation are often part of the scenario.

Cannabis therapy can assist in a myriad of ways, from treating symptoms like anxiety, insomnia, and bulimia, to enhancing the effects of other mental and spiritual therapies. Although every case has been extremely complex, with many layers of issues, I have successfully treated several clients with PTSD using holistic therapy. They ranged from victims of war to immigrants persecuted during their travels to sexual or domestic abuse victims. After intense and long-term therapy, they were able to heal a great deal. Below is one soldier's story.

James's Story

James is a Marine Corps veteran who served two tours in Iraq, where he was on an infantry assault team from 2004 to 2008. For two years after his return, he was haunted by flashback nightmares. He would wake up sweating, shouting, disoriented, and could not go back to sleep. He then played hours of video games and became severely sleep deprived. James also suffered frequent migraines related to a bomb that went off near his vehicle. He overreacted to loud noises and sudden unexpected movements. He felt "on alert" yet exhausted all the time. He was so short-tempered and combative that he kept getting fired from jobs and could no longer live with his girlfriend. The antidepressants, opiates, sedatives, amphetamines, and mood stabilizers prescribed by his Department of Veterans Affairs (VA) doctors left him feeling disconnected from people and unable to think clearly or feel anything. He called them his "zombie cocktail," but they did not subdue the nightmares or his outbursts. When I met James, he was living in his parents' basement while waiting for admission to an inpatient PTSD clinic run by the VA. He called me from Arizona, where they had recently legalized medical marijuana, and we began to work together over the phone.

James began his cannabis therapy by smoking a joint with a 4:1 ratio of CBD:THC. For the first time since returning from combat he was able to relax. "I didn't even need to play video games," he said in surprise. "I was content to just sit on the couch and watch the birds out the window . . . for two hours!" He smoked these joints whenever irritable and within three weeks found that with them and breathing *exercises, he could get through most days without an outburst or argument. However, he still wasn't sleeping and the nightmares had not been reduced. He slowly reduced his "one pot a day" coffee intake to zero and added herbal teas and nervines like oat seed, chamomile, and passionflower before we decided to up his dose of THC before bed in the form of a THC-rich marijuana cookie. The first night, he slept five hours straight with no nightmares and woke up feeling rested for the first time in five years. "I couldn't believe it! Cured by a cookie? My doctors would think I was nuts!" So, he did not tell them. He was soon sleeping through seven nights out of ten. "I felt like a whole new person—new energy, a whole new outlook on life." At this point we began to have regular therapy sessions over the phone. Over the next two years, he was able to wean himself off the "zombie cocktail" except for occasional opiates for his less frequent but still occurring migraines. He has held down a job as a medic for the past six months and is making plans to move into his own apartment. His parents and his girlfriend have stuck with him, and they feel that he is getting back to his old self—his pre-PTSD self.*

NON-ANXIETY-BASED CONDITIONS

Autism Spectrum Disorder

The U.S. Centers for Disease Control (CDC) estimates that one in sixty-eight American kids is on the autism spectrum. Autism spectrum disorder refers to a range of conditions characterized by lack of social skills, repetitive behaviors, and difficulties with or absence of speech and forms of nonverbal communication. Autistic people process sensory information differently, and thus they already live with an "altered perception of reality" in which everyday sensory input can be overwhelming. Some find comfort in routine and in repetitive motions like rocking or hand flapping. Although it impairs the ability to communicate and interact, and other symptoms can be debilitating, autism also often includes unique abilities and talents. Good statistics are unavailable, but experts estimate that one in ten autistic people demonstrates a savant talent and that over half of all savants are autistic.[10]

Bonni Goldstein, M.D., a cannabis clinician, pediatrician, and author of *Cannabis Revealed,* hypothesizes that a disruption in the ECS may be a contributing factor to the development of autism.[11] Mice and rat studies have found a connection with the gene causing fragile X syndrome, which is involved in some autism disorders and also causes an abnormal ECS.[12] An increased number of cannabinoid receptors have been found in the white blood cells of children with autism, indicating that their bodies are searching for cannabinoids. Marijuana medicine can normalize this defect and correct behavioral abnormalities.

Pediatricians, physicians, and parents who administer cannabis therapy for autism report reductions in the frequency and severity of tantrums, rage, self-injury, anxiety, sleep disturbances, and property destruction. They also witness increased happiness and ability to learn as well as more flexibility and tolerance for interruption of routine.

In one study, CBD was given to fifty-three autistic children for two months. Improvement was seen in symptoms for most. "Self-injury and rage attacks improved in 67.6% and worsened in 8.8%. Hyperactivity symptoms improved in 68.4%, did not change in 28.9% and worsened in 2.6%. Sleep problems improved in 71.4% and worsened in 4.7%. Anxiety improved in 47.1% and worsened in 23.5%. Adverse effects, mostly somnolence and change in appetite, were mild."[13]

Mason's Story

Lisa's twelve-year-old son, Mason, is severely autistic. He was diagnosed at age two. She describes their trajectory toward cannabis therapy: "At eighteen months, we started to notice huge changes in his behavior. Up until then he was loving, affectionate, and laughed a lot. Then he just stopped interacting with us. He wouldn't make eye contact and stopped playing with his older brother. He would only eat yellow food. He seemed not to hear us. He started bouncing on the trampoline all the time, day and night. He wouldn't speak and seemed to have lost the few words he had learned. Then he had a seizure, and then another one. We were going to the hospital regularly. He started hitting himself and would have terrible tantrums all the time. We were at wit's end. It was a nightmare."

After the diagnosis Lisa and her husband, Stan, tried many of the recommended vocal and behavioral therapies. They did not see much change in their child, and the therapies were too expensive for them to continue after the first three years. Mason tried the usual prescribed medications, including antidepressants, antianxiety medications, and eventually antipsychotic drugs. The side effects included involuntary movements, anxiety, weight gain, nausea, constipation, headaches, dizziness, fatigue, and insomnia. Some medications turned the child into a zombie and others caused his tantrums to increase.

"As he grew larger and angrier he was harder to handle and it was harder to protect him from himself. We didn't know what to do anymore. We didn't know if we were going to be able to keep him at home."

This was about the time that CBD was becoming known for childhood seizures and Lisa heard about it from a friend. She called me to see if it might help Mason's seizures. We discussed using whole plant medicine instead of isolated CBD, and how it might help with his other symptoms too. She decided to try a concentrated CBD oil that was 18:1 CBD:THC and included roots.

"I gave him the first dose and it was like a miracle! He became calmer, less anxious, and less violent. He was more attentive to his therapists and would look at me when I spoke to him. Then he started talking! In the first two months of cannabis oil, he said hundreds of words. He began playing with his little sister and eating everything in sight. Cannabis oil certainly did not cure his autism entirely, but it was a game changer for my whole family."

Not stymied by politics, scientists in other countries, like Spain and Israel, are reporting significant benefits in treating these disorders with cannabis. Israeli researchers, including Raphael Mechoulam, the discoverer of THC and the endocannabinoid system, have shown that cannabis is a beneficial treatment for children. They found cannabis to be a safe and effective option to relieve common symptoms like seizures, tics, depression, restlessness, and rage attacks. One study reported that after six months of cannabis treatment 80 percent of 188 participants on the autism spectrum reported some level of improvement, including in quality of life and positive mood; 43 percent reported improved ability to shower and dress independently.[14]

Unlike the pharmaceutical medications often prescribed for treating autism symptoms, pot offers "conduct-normalizing" effects without sedation. Patients remain alert but not anxious. Patients acquire skills they had either lost or never had, like speaking, interacting with a tablet, or listening to music. Patients may even give hugs—in many cases parents receive the first affection they have had from their child since they were a toddler. Many children with an autism spectrum disorder seem unhappy and to be in constant pain or suffering. Perhaps they are frustrated with not being able to communicate. With simple weed some children smile or even laugh for the first time! These changes might seem trivial, but for the children's parents, they are major breakthroughs. Cannabis therapy offers some hope without harm, where none has previously existed. Often there is improvement with the first dose, so parents and caregivers might know immediately if cannabis is the right medicine for their charges.[15]

Cannabis therapy also benefits the parents and caregivers of special needs children and adults. According to Marian Fry, M.D., pot-smoking patients with parenting problems saw an "enhanced flexibility and an ability to identify the child's needs as those of a separate and unique individual . . .The parent becomes present and the child benefits from the increased positive attention . . . Patients say cannabis makes them less self-centered and egocentric and more aware of the needs of other people."[16]

Schizophrenia and Psychosis

> *Madness is a journey of self-discovery, which can bring spiritual enlightenment.*
>
> R. D. LAING*

One of the most enduring myths surrounding pot is that it causes schizophrenia. This is untrue. A profound ignorance still exists as to the molecular mechanisms behind schizophrenia. Not only is weed not a trigger for schizophrenia, in some cases it can be a successful treatment. Schizophrenia is a serious, complex, long-term condition that interferes with a person's ability to think clearly, manage emotions, make decisions, and relate to others. Although schizophrenia can occur at any age, the average age of onset tends to be in the late teens to the early twenties for men, and the late twenties to early thirties for women. Symptoms may include hallucinations; delusions; being emotionally flat or speaking in a dull, disconnected way; and organizational and cognitive difficulties. Often individuals are unaware that they have the illness. Many patients reject pharmaceutical antipsychotic treatments due to their extremely strong side effects, which include motor impairment, weight gain, and zombification as well as permanent damage to the kidneys and other organs.

Patients with schizophrenia have enhanced levels of endogenous cannabinoids in their blood and cerebrospinal fluid. Neuroimaging studies and postmortem examinations have shown that they also have increased levels of cannabinoid receptors in their brains. At the behavioral level, people with schizophrenia often have elevated rates of pot smoking. Those who self-report tend to prefer leaf or trim over bud, finding the strength of bud overwhelming. This indicates that too much THC, with its anxiogenic properties, might aggravate their psychic difficulties.

---

*R. D. Laing was a Scottish psychiatrist who wrote extensively on the experience of psychosis. His seminal work, *The Divided Self: An Existential Study in Sanity and Madness*, was written when he was just twenty-eight years old and published in 1960. It became a bestseller and earned him a global reputation. His experimental no-locks and no-medication asylum and his striking ability to think outside the conventional box revolutionized the treatment of psychosis and schizophrenia throughout Great Britain.

CBD has antipsychotic and relaxing properties and modulates the psychoactive properties of THC. Given the increased rates of cannabis use among people with schizophrenia, along with the role of the endocannabinoid system in the pathophysiology of the disease, I believe that consuming CBD, which will have a longer lasting effect than smoking it, will be a more popular choice for those who self-medicate for these disorders.

To summarize: the limited information available about the effects of cannabis therapy for schizophrenics comes down to two points. There is no valid evidence that marijuana causes schizophrenia, and schizophrenics who self-medicate with pot seem to prefer low-THC medicines.

A Spiritual Component: Schizophrenic or Shaman?

It is useful to note here that what Westerners diagnose as psychotic or schizophrenic disorders is celebrated in other cultures as a call into shamanism. "Psychotic-like" behaviors and thinking mirror those of indigenous shamans who communicate with spirits that others cannot sense. Shamans and schizophrenics "keep a foot in both worlds" to act as a bridge between spirits and the community.

According to American ethnobotanist Terence McKenna, "What is called the initiatory crisis in shamanism is nothing more than a schizophrenic break with ordinary reality. To become schizophrenic is a wonderful, wonderful opportunity. The trick is to make sure that you're nowhere where straight people can get at you." He also noted, "A shaman is someone who swims in the same ocean as the schizophrenic, but the shaman has thousands and thousands of years of sanctioned technique and tradition to draw upon. In a traditional society, if you exhibited 'schizophrenic' tendencies, you are immediately drawn out of the pack and put under the care and tutelage of master shamans."[17]

Malidoma Somé, Ph.D., a West African shaman who came to the United States for graduate studies in mental health, was interviewed by Stephanie Marohn, author of The Natural Medicine Guide to Schizophrenia. Somé observed that, "What those in the West view as mental illness, the

Dagara people regard as good news from the other world. The person going through the crisis has been chosen as a medium for a message to the community that needs to be communicated from the spirit realm."[18]

Attention Deficit Hyperactivity Disorder (ADHD)

Attention deficit hyperactivity disorder is a chronic condition characterized by difficulties with concentration and focus, hyperactivity, and impulsiveness. (This should absolutely not be confused with normal activities of childhood.) There are three recognized types of ADHD: inattentive, hyperactive/impulsive, and combined.

Cannabis slows down the rate of attentional shift and increases the span and intensity of concentration. One paper published in 1991 by the Department of Psychiatry and Behavioral Sciences at George Washington Medical Center reported:

Absorption (a trait capacity for total attentional involvement) was reported to increase during episodes of marijuana intoxication. . . Additionally, within the drug-using group, a positive correlation between frequency of marijuana use and affective ratings of these experiences was found. The findings support the hypothesis that a specific type of alteration in consciousness that enhances capacity for total attentional involvement (absorption) characterizes marijuana intoxication, and that this enhancement may act as a reinforcement, possibly influencing future use.[19]

Cannabis competes with dopamine at receptor sites and inhibits the speed of nerve transmission. Parents report seeing an immediate shift in their children "from fidget to focus." Grades go up, relationships improve, and their children are happier. Being high helps those with ADHD to filter out distractions and focus on one thing at a time. It also helps people clearly see what is the most essential thing for them, personally, to focus on. People who use marijuana literally spend more time with each thought, giving them time to process the thoughts and feel the emotions attached to them.

The two most commonly prescribed drugs for adults and children with ADHD, Adderall and Ritalin, are dangerously addictive amphetamines, or speed. These sympathomimetic drugs (also known as adrenergic drugs) stimulate the sympathetic nervous system. When a tolerance builds up, users are unable to function without higher and higher doses. "Amphetamine prescriptions, primarily Adderall, have increased dramatically recently, from 1.3 million in 1996 to nearly 6 million in 1999."[20]

Drug recovery centers see the resulting methamphetamine addictions every day: "The street value of Adderall is significant, and those who develop addictions to this specific prescription might eventually turn to a cheaper and more readily available alternative. Unfortunately, the alternative to prescription amphetamines is often methamphetamine."[21]

In 2017 a reported 964,000 people aged twelve or older had meth problems, up from 684,000 in 2016.[22]

Although the information is not tracked, it appears as if the United States now has a huge problem with adult speed addicts who began with childhood prescriptions of Adderall. I have clients who began chopping and snorting their Ritalin by age eleven and moved on to street methamphetamine when their pediatricians stopped providing it—all because they couldn't sit still in school. Amphetamines can permanently damage and even destroy the nervous system and are notoriously difficult to kick.

Pot, on the other hand, is neuroprotective and can also help addicts heal from their addiction. For those who choose to continue using these speedy drugs, cannabis can help alleviate the side effects like difficulty sleeping, depressed appetite, and jitteriness.

Depression

Depression is expressed as an utter lack of energy and emotion; listlessness about life; a downtrodden and narrow perspective on one's personal situation; and an absence of inspiration, joy, motivation, and other emotions. Depression often manifests as overall exhaustion caused by suppressing emotions, "filtering out" chronic pain, or suppressing or obsessing on trauma. It takes a huge amount of energy for a person to ignore and suppress.

Here's how actor Jim Carrey characterized depression:

This is all ego: desiring to be important, to be someone, to matter. In reality, this grasping at a singular identity brings us only pain and suffering, for three main reasons. One, it introduces a separation between us and all other beings that dishonors our inherent, interconnected nature. Two, it deludes us into thinking that things are not supposed to change—that we are not supposed to change. Three, it leads us away from resting in our own basic goodness, as it makes us feel that we aren't enough just as we are, right now. Depression is your body saying fuck you, I don't want to be this character anymore, I don't want to hold up this avatar that you've created in the world. It's too much for me. You should think of the word "depressed" as "deep rest." Your body needs to be depressed. It needs deep rest from the character that you've been trying to play.[23]

Be aware that depression is often confused with sadness or grief. Sadness and grief are natural emotions and should not be medicated. Emotions need to be experienced as they come up, not repressed so that a patient can "get on with their life." People feel sluggish or "underwater" while experiencing grief because the thyroid gland naturally slows metabolism by half so that a person can slow down and heal.

Dozens of studies and even human trials have confirmed the natural antidepressant and mood-elevating effects of cannabis, potentially by enhancing CB1 activity in the hippocampus. It literally lifts the spirit. Cannabis has been found to be more effective in treating depression than standard prescriptions and over-the-counter medications, and without harmful side effects. This is because marijuana helps us bring up what has been bottled up and examine it without fear, shame, or loathing. People can find acceptance and compassion for themselves as their outlook becomes fuller, broader, and more energized. It also brings us clearer insight into predicaments and relationships and helps one stay in the present and avoid obsessing on memories of difficult times.

Everyone's depression is different, but a combination of cannabis therapy, nervine and adaptogenic herbs, counseling, exercise, and massage can improve anyone's depression.

> *Warning:* Pharmaceutical antidepressant drugs can increase thoughts of and attempts at suicide and homicide. The FDA now mandates black box labels on these drugs, the strongest warning label there is. There are many reports and studies confirming that SSRI antidepressants can cause violence, suicide, mania, and other forms of psychotic and bizarre behavior.[24]

"Since the Columbine massacre, there have been 31 documented mass shootings in the United States of America. The two constant variables that remained were that the vast majority of shooters had been formally diagnosed with a mental illness and were prescribed psychiatric medications."[25]

Nearly every mass shooter in the last twenty years was using a prescription psychotropic drug? I wish we knew how many used cannabis.

Alzheimer's Disease

Alzheimer's disease accounts for 60 to 80 percent of dementia cases in the elderly. Doctors diagnose the disease from a broad symptom profile that includes cognitive decline, behavioral changes, mood changes, depression, paranoia, loss of appetite, and difficulty with muscle control. With time, the symptoms increase in severity and reduce a person's ability to perform everyday activities.

Alzheimer's patients demonstrate abnormal functioning of their endocannabinoid system. This leads to a buildup of amyloid plaque in the brain as well as the disfigurement of a protein called *tau,* which prevents delivery of nutrients to brain cells and induces inflammation.[26]

Cannabis is an ideal therapy for Alzheimer's disease for a multitude of reasons. First, it can cross the blood-brain barrier and act as a neuroprotectant and anti-inflammatory in the brain. Second, it inhibits acetylcholinesterase from breaking down the "memory molecule" acetylcholine. Third, it prevents tau proteins from creating plaque. Fourth, it neutralizes existing plaque buildup by disrupting the twisting and resulting clumping of tau proteins and is 80 percent better at this than the existing prescription drugs.[27]

The Canadian Agency for Drugs and Technologies in Health has found evidence suggesting that "medical cannabis may be effective for treating agitation, disinhibition, irritability, aberrant motor behaviour, and nocturnal behaviour disorders as well as aberrant vocalization and resting care, which are neuropsychiatric symptoms associated with dementia. There was also limited evidence of improvement in rigidity and cognitive scores as assessed by Mini-Mental State Examination."[28]

Dr. Jeffrey Hergenrather,* a cannabis clinician in Northern California with decades of experience, has seen these effects in action. At the urging of a staff nurse who had recently lost another patient to the dangerous black box drugs, Dr. Hergenrather and the staff psychiatrist developed a cannabis therapy plan for every patient in the facility and saw immediate, significant results. They monitored patients for the multiple symptoms associated with dementia and found improvements of *all* symptoms in *all* the patients. Patients experienced decreased agitation, aggression, self-mutilation, and pain and increased appetite, sleep quality, and mood. Most were taken off black box prescriptions and the rest used far less than before.[29] Dr. Hergenrather starts new patients with 10 mg of THC and 10 mg of CBD twice a day. Then he adjusts the dosages upward until the desired results are achieved for each patient.

Studies indicate that in treating Alzheimer's, whole plant medicines have a huge advantage over isolated or synthetic cannabinoids. According to Dr. Ethan Russo,

Based on its pharmacology, cannabis components may provide myriad benefits on target symptoms in this complex disorder:

---

*Now retired, cannabis consultation physician Jeffrey Hergenrather is a former president of the Society of Cannabis Clinicians, which produces, among other things, *O'Shaughnessy's: The Journal of Cannabis in Clinical Practice.* He is a member of the International Cannabinoid Research Society and the International Association of Cannabinoid Medicine. In his current general practice, he is focusing his research on inflammatory bowel disease, Alzheimer's disease, and dementia.

Agitation: THC, CBD, linalool

Psychosis: CBD

Insomnia/Restlessness: THC, linalool

Anorexia: THC

Aggression: THC, CBD, linalool

Depression: THC, limonene, CBD

Pain: THC, CBD

Memory: alpha-pinene (Russo, 2011; Russo and Marcu, 2017), THC

Neuroprotection: CBD, THC

Reduced Aβ plaque formation: THC, CBD, THCA

Thus, an extract of a Type II chemovar of cannabis (THC/CBD) with a sufficient pinene fraction would seem to be an excellent candidate.[30]

ADDICTION DISORDERS

Alcoholism

Marijuana helps addicts in many ways, including harm reduction through substitution, management of symptoms like anxiety or pain that led to the addiction, withdrawal symptom management, and healing the addiction itself.

There are ample historical references to American and European physicians using cannabis to treat alcohol and opiate addiction. Standard U.S. medical texts at the turn of the nineteenth century listed cannabis as a treatment for the delirium tremens ("the shakes") associated with advanced alcoholism. In 1953, physicians Thompson and Proctor used synthetic THC in the treatment of alcohol withdrawal and reported that symptoms including tremulousness, restlessness, apprehension, and anorexia were ameliorated in 84 percent of treated patients. One subject in the study also had a history of schizophrenia. On the second day of alcohol withdrawal, before THC was administered, he became agitated, fearful, restless, and slept poorly. This became worse on the third day when he appeared disoriented as to time and place, exhibited mood swings, chewed his fingernails, cried, and was unable to swallow.

These symptoms disappeared for a five-hour period after the THC was administered.[31]

Farther back in history we find notes left by physicians prescribing cannabis. One Dr. Kane, in 1881, described a patient who successfully took hashish to control her alcohol addiction. In the same era, a Dr. Birch weaned a patient off alcohol by using opiates, causing the patient to become addicted to them. Then they were prescribed cannabis to get off the opiates.[32]

In 1873, the Indian Government Finance Department Resolution recommended against suppressing cannabis use for fear that people "would in all probability have recourse to some other stimulant such as alcohol." The Indian Hemp Drugs Commission Report of 1894 articulated the same concern, writing that reducing access to cannabis would have the effect of "driving the consumers to have recourse to other stimulants or narcotics which may be more deleterious."[33]

In more modern times, in 2004 Dr. Tod Hiro Mikuriya* published a study of ninety-two patients for whom he had prescribed cannabis as a treatment for their alcohol or drug dependence.[34] All of them found it "very effective" or "effective." Nine patients achieved total abstinence from alcohol and attributed their success to cannabis. They reported periods of abstinence ranging from two to nineteen years. They liked pot because it had no harmful side effects, was better at managing their symptoms, and because it had no withdrawal problems. Twenty-nine reported that they had formerly used alcohol for pain relief and were now using cannabis instead. Forty-four reported that they had previously used alcohol to

---

*Tod Hiro Mikuriya was a psychiatrist and the director of nonclassified marijuana research for the National Institute of Mental Health Center for Narcotics and Drug Abuse Studies in 1967. His 1972 self-published book *Marijuana Medical Papers 1839–1972* became a landmark in the modern movement for the legalization of medical marijuana. Until his death in May 2007, he continued in private psychiatric practice limited to cannabis clinical consultation. He prescribed marijuana for over nine thousand patients. In 1999, Mikuriya founded the California Cannabis Research Medical Group (CCRMG) to help physicians share and exchange data about cannabis use by their patients. In 2004 the CCRMG formed the Society of Cannabis Clinicians (SCC) to facilitate voluntary medical standards for physician-approved cannabis.

medicate mood disorders such as depression, anxiety, stress, or PTSD and that marijuana relieved these issues better than alcohol.

Patients who discontinued pot use reported a return of symptoms, listed below.

"I crave alcohol when I can't smoke marijuana."

"I started drinking a lot more."

"More anxiety, less happiness."

"I quit using cannabis while I was in the army and my drinking doubled. I was also involved in several violent incidents due to alcohol."

"My caretaker got arrested and I lived too far from the city to purchase at a club, and I started doing heroin again and almost killed myself and some of my friends."

"Alcohol consumption increases and so does depression."

Three patients reported a sad irony: they had "fallen off the wagon" when they had to stop using cannabis in anticipation of drug tests or because they were in a treatment program.

Because abstinence-only support groups like Alcoholics Anonymous are not all that successful (more than 60 percent of patients relapse), Mikuriya suggested the development of groups tailored toward those who wish to use cannabis during recovery.

Another study, this one from the University of British Columbia, found that "addicts can benefit from using marijuana to heal their addictions." Zach Walsh, Ph.D., UBC associate professor and lead researcher in the study, observes that "people are using cannabis as an exit drug to reduce use of substances that are more harmful, such as opioid pain medication." The team also found evidence that cannabis could be helpful in treating the symptoms of social anxiety, PTSD, and depression.[35]

But perhaps Dr. Mikuriya put it best:

It would appear that for selected alcoholics the substitution of smoked cannabis for alcohol may be of marked rehabilitative value. In the experience of certain alcoholics, cannabis use is discovered to overcome pain and depression, target conditions for which alcohol is originally used, but without the disinhibited emotions or the physiologic damage. By substituting cannabis for alcohol, patients were able to reduce the harm their intoxication caused themselves and others.

He goes on to explain how prescribing cannabis makes him a better doctor:

As a certified addictionologist, I have supervised both inpatient and outpatient treatment for thousands of patients since 1969. In the traditional alcoholism medical-treatment model, the physician is an authority figure to a patient whose life has spun out of control. The patient enters under coercive circumstances, frequently under court order, with physiologies in toxic disarray. After detoxification the patient leaves, usually with powers of denial intact.

Treating alcoholism by cannabis substitution creates a different doctor-patient relationship. My most important service is to end their criminal status, which often brings an expression of relief. An alliance is created that promotes candor and trust. The physician is permitted to act as a coach or an enabler in a positive sense. As enumerated by patients, the benefits can be profound: self-respect is enhanced; family and community relationships improve; a sense of social alienation diminishes. A recurrent theme at follow-up visits is the developing sense of freedom as cannabis use replaces the intoxication-withdrawal-recovery cycle, freedom to look into the future and plan instead of being mired in a dysfunctional past and present, and freedom from crisis and distraction, making possible pursuit of long-term goals that include family and community.[36]

So not only is weed not a gateway to drug addiction, it can be a cure. It is a healthy substitute for addictive drugs or addictive behaviors. It aids and, in some cases, eliminates withdrawal symptoms. It leads to a trusting relationship between doctors and patients. It furthers psychological health by improving sleep, respiration, appetite, and nutrient absorption. It balances the ANS. It relieves the physical pain for which many addicts use other drugs. It aids in relieving stress and helping the body adapt to a new chemistry. Even more importantly, cannabis therapy also helps one face and examine the unconscious problems and motives behind the addiction, leading to relief of the stress and depression that are often at its roots.

Barbara's Story

At age sixty-one Barbara had knee replacement surgery. Her doctors sent her home with prescriptions for opiates to control the pain while it healed. She lived alone and had to "get back on her feet" sooner than recommended. "The pain was pretty intense, but manageable with the pain pills. Except at night. My knee would just throb and keep me up all night. So I started taking an extra dose when I would wake up. Then I tried an extra dose before bed, too, so I could fall asleep. I ran through those pills pretty quick. I was also still constipated even a few weeks after the surgery."

Her doctor renewed her prescription and warned her to reduce the amount she was using. She tried, but the pain and insomnia made it very difficult. Also, she now had lower back pain due to her limp. This was about the time she came to me for help, saying, "My doctor refused to re-up my prescription, and now I don't know what I am going to do!"

I discussed many options with her, and she decided that a slow withdrawal from the opiates and counseling for pain management would be the best method for her. She started a high dose of an herbal medicine called kratom, which works via the same pain-blocking opiate receptors that the prescription pills use. She started a gentle, whole plant cannabis medicine at the same time, and she began doing breathing exercises when the pain seemed the worst. We treated her back pain with bodywork and a cannabis topical salve.

The first week she reduced her prescription opiate by 25 percent and increased her cannabis dose by the same amount. I taught her some pain control meditations that she did before each dose of medicine. She began hydrotherapy (repeatedly alternating hot and cold compresses) on the knee, followed by a topical cannabis salve. She began herbal therapy for constipation.

The second week, she decreased her prescription dose another 25 percent, reduced her kratom dose by 25 percent, and increased her cannabis by 25 percent. The pain was quite manageable during the day now, and she was not feeling "grumpy," as she had when she'd tried to reduce her prescription medication. She was having more frequent bowel movements.

The third week she ceased using the prescription during the day, reduced her kratom dosage by another 25 percent, and increased her cannabis dose by 25 percent. By the fourth week, she was off the prescription opiates entirely and no longer constipated. A week later, she ceased using the kratom.

Barbara remains on a maintenance dose of cannabis to prevent a recurrence of a previous cancer. Her knee pain is now only occasional, and she treats it with hydrotherapy and the cannabis salve.

Opioid Addiction

The statistics are astounding. Opioid abuse is a problem for more than two million Americans and fifteen million people worldwide. This number does not include the problems that addicts cause for the people around them, the medical system, or the economy.

This addiction kills more than forty-seven thousand Americans a year. That is over nine hundred a week. If this were a virus, they would call in the CDC! But it's not, and more than 40 percent of overdoses are from prescription opioids, including Vicodin, OxyContin, Percocet, codeine, morphine, and fentanyl. The rest are from heroin. Many heroin addictions start with addictions to prescribed pharmaceuticals.

One might conclude that this is an epidemic that is sanctioned by the state, the AMA, and the pharmaceutical corporations. Their recommendation for opioid addiction is another prescription opioid, methadone. They call it a "safe treatment" for opiate addiction when used under medical supervision and in conjunction with therapy. Once addicts begin taking methadone, they must take it on a long-term basis. If they want to quit methadone, they will have to be safely weaned off it under medical supervision. According to Harvard Medical School, only 25 percent of people admitted to a methadone "maintenance" program will be able to quit. Another 25 percent will have to continue using methadone as a replacement medication. The rest remain addicted to opioids.[37] Not a great success rate.

Methadone has mild side effects like stomach pain, constipation, and sweating but also has more severe side effects like slowed breathing, sexual dysfunction, nausea, vomiting, restlessness, and itchy skin. Long-term side effects of methadone include lung and respiratory problems. Combining methadone with sedatives, depressants, or alcohol can result in depressed breathing, unconsciousness, coma, and death.

If an addict quits methadone, or any opioid, "cold turkey," he or she can expect high anxiety, extreme pain, restlessness, muscle cramps and spasms, muscle, bone, and nerve pain, insomnia, diarrhea, vomiting, cold flashes with goosebumps, and involuntary leg movements. Major withdrawal symptoms peak between twenty-four and forty-eight hours after the last dose and subside after about a week for most. However, for some people they can last for many months.

On the other hand, a treatment using cannabis therapy improves the health of the addict, has no side effects, and is extremely safe to use.

Cannabis therapy potentiates opiates, so people can begin reducing their dosages of opioids immediately and continue to reduce their dosage without side effects or the need for medical supervision. Most users can cut their opioid intake by 75 to 100 percent by using weed, making the Queen of Herbs a more powerful antidote for opiate addiction than any other medication. A 2014 study published in *JAMA Internal Medicine* examined data between 1999 and 2010 and found that states with medical marijuana laws had a 25 percent lower annual opioid overdose death rate compared to states without such laws.[38]

If someone wants to quit an opioid cold turkey, cannabis will reduce the withdrawal symptoms and make them bearable as well as help with anxiety, depression, pain, muscle spasms, and mood. She will also rebalance the neurotransmitters that are knocked out of production with opioid addiction and thus improve mood and general suffering. She can also provide a much safer therapy for whatever caused the addict to initially start using opiates.

Anita Willard Briscoe, a psychiatric nurse practitioner with a private practice in Albuquerque, New Mexico, teamed up with two others in her field and a psychiatrist to collect self-reported data from four hundred opioid-addicted patients. Twenty-five percent reported being able to quit opioids using marijuana alone. According to Briscoe:

> They state it calms down their cravings, relaxes their . . . anxiety and is helping to keep them off opioids. . . . If they are in pain, cannabis is helping relieve their pain, often to the point that they don't need opiates anymore. [Medical marijuana] will help the state's children if the parents aren't hooked on prescription pills and heroin. It will help our economy, because they will get on their feet and get jobs. Crime will go down. This is a simple solution to our heroin problem. There is no reason not to sign off on this.[39]

When Joe Schrank, a social worker who has worked at various detox centers and clean houses throughout Los Angeles, started recommending pot for addicts, the results were so rewarding he found himself asking, "Why didn't we do this years ago? One of the barriers in entry to treatment is detox. Many people are afraid of it. It's difficult to break this step. But when they're told, 'Hey, you can smoke pot,' it softens the blow."[40]

Clearly, an addiction that affects fifteen million people worldwide and kills more than nine hundred Americans a week is an epidemic. No matter the cause or who is at fault, we must try everything in our power to rectify the situation. Why not try marijuana? The answer may be in Dr. Grinspoon's observation that "there is something very special about illicit drugs. If they don't always make the drug user behave irrationally, they certainly cause many non-users to behave that way."[41]

The Tobacco Epidemic

The World Health Organization estimates 8 million deaths a year in the world due to tobacco abuse, 1.2 million of which are due to second-hand smoke. Tobacco addiction is also one of the biggest contributors to poverty in low and middle-income countries. The current prevalence of electronic cigarettes, often more poisonous than commercial cigarettes, has increased addiction problems and deaths worldwide.

The WHO claims that among those aware of tobacco's health risks, most want to quit and that counseling and medication can more than double the chance of quitting successfully. I don't know what medication WHO is referring to, but cannabis can certainly help people quit tobacco. By substituting cannabis joints, pipes, or safe vaporizing for tobacco cigarettes, the intake of harmful chemicals is immediately reduced and prevention and treatment of any lung cancers or other diseases can begin.

Pot can help people slowly reduce their tobacco intake by making blends that are at first high tobacco/low cannabis and then working toward high cannabis/low tobacco blends. This helps the body adjust slowly and reduces or eliminates tobacco withdrawal symptoms.

High-CBD cannabis in any form (except topical) will calm and rebalance the addict's nervous system while they are quitting and will reduce inflammation in the lungs. (See also the anxiety section in this chapter.)

Although tobacco addiction, unlike most other drug and alcohol addictions, is not always a direct result of mental or spiritual imbalance, gaining a deeper understanding of oneself in the process of quitting can only be beneficial. THC cannabis can help this process.

I am excited to bring this information to the public because the American health system offers such a sad lack of mental health support, especially in the realm of anxiety, addiction, and depression disorders that are sweeping our country. Unlike harmful prescription psych medicines, here we have an ally in nature that can truly help us with autism, psychosis, ADHD, and Alzheimer's disease. Mary Jane is available to help us and maintain our mental health and spiritual connection. So, you see, getting high is good for you.

5

Physical Systems and Conditions That Benefit from Cannabis

The Marijuana Medical Handbook: Practical Guide to Therapeutic Uses of Marijuana, written by Ed Rosenthal,* Dale Gieringer†, and Dr. Gregory Carter‡, lists a total of 240 diseases and conditions that benefit from marijuana therapy. I will not discuss all 240 here, but we will look at each of the body's systems and how they are regulated by

---

*Ed Rosenthal is the world's leading expert on the cultivation of marijuana and a prolific author, publisher, and advocate for the legalization of marijuana. He served as a columnist for *High Times Magazine* during the 1980s and 1990s. His other books include *Marijuana Grower's Handbook, The Big Book of Buds, Medical Marijuana 101,* and many more.

†Dale Gieringer, Ph.D., has been the state coordinator of California's National Organization for the Reform of Marijuana Laws (NORML) since 1987. He received his Ph.D. at Stanford on the topic of DEA drug regulation. He is the author of articles on marijuana and driving safety, drug testing, marijuana health mythology, the economics of marijuana legalization, and DEA "drug enforcement abuse." He was one of the original coauthors of California's medical marijuana initiative, Prop. 215, and a proponent of Oakland's Measure Z cannabis initiative in 2004. In 2010, he was named *High Times* Freedom Fighter of the Year.

‡Gregory T. Carter, M.D., is a founding member of the American Board of Neuromuscular Medicine. He currently serves as chief medical officer at St. Luke's Rehabilitation Institute in Washington and is clinical professor of medical education and clinical sciences at Washington State University.

the endocannabinoid system and thereby can benefit from cannabis therapy. I will describe the role of ganja in prevention and treatment of cancer and mental and spiritual conditions. I end with a list of symptoms that weed can relieve.

BODY SYSTEMS

The Reproductive System

Both the male and female reproductive systems are regulated by the endocannabinoid system (ECS), which was introduced in detail in chapter 1. Reproductive organs like the uterus and testes manufacture cannabinoids to control hormones, fertility, implantation of fertilized eggs, and development of the embryo. For example, cannabinoids can slow down hormone production, and hormones modulate protein expression in the ECS. These cannabinoids also control inflammation.

In females, low levels of the endocannabinoid anandamide are associated with menstrual dysfunction, infertility, poor neurochemical communication between mother and fetus, morning sickness, and failure to thrive syndrome. In males, cannabinoids regulate spermatogenesis, erections, and fertility. One could surmise that a deficient ECS would cause problems in these areas. However, there is not much research, and, aside from cancers, most of my own experience with cannabis and reproductive disorders comes anecdotally from female clients; so, that is what I have to offer here.

Many reproductive problems can be alleviated with whole plant cannabis supplementation. For example, many women find relief from menstrual cramps by smoking leaves or flowers. Others find relief by using cannabis vaginal suppositories. Sore breasts can be massaged with topicals. Digestive distress can be calmed with cannabis tea. The analgesic, anti-inflammatory, antispasmodic, and hormone-balancing qualities of cannabis contribute to their relief and so do the relaxing and sleep-inducing qualities of the medicine. Many women who suffer from premenstrual symptoms are deficient in gamma-linoleic acid (GLA) and find relief with daily doses of 5 ml of hemp seed oil, which contains 150–200 mg of GLA.

Women find emotional and psychological relief from cannabis as well as relief from physical symptoms. Women evolved to "multitask"—to raise children and run families. Traditionally, during menstruation, women were relieved of their responsibilities and went to places where they could be still to allow their inflamed uterine muscle to do her work, quiet places so as to hear their own thoughts and be in the company of other women who are in the same situation.

Today, women have forgotten this, and we continue living our busy lives right through our cycle, without pause to process and rest. When events and emotions pop up needing our attention, we have learned to ignore them. This leads to issues building up and can cause us to be emotionally unstable, short-tempered, and easily frustrated. We blame it on our "hormones," but in fact it is due to ignoring what the hormones are inducing us to do—be still and quiet, and process. Because Mary Jane helps us to relax and focus, she can be a vital part of a monthly ritual to relax, take care of our own needs, rebalance our hormones, and process our emotions. I have met with countless women who have cured their PMS with a monthly dose of marijuana and a hot bath, sauna, creative activity, or meditation.

Weed has an ancient history as an aphrodisiac that can help immediately or bring sexual health over time. She has the characteristics of both a psychological and a physiological sexual booster, as she can relax muscles, increase blood flow, and balance hormone levels. She can also increase focus and remove the unconscious defense mechanisms that hinder intimacy. In this realm, pot can be dose dependent, with small doses stimulating but large doses sedating. She works differently with each individual but is completely safe to experiment with. She's not just for internal use: many of my clients love cannabis infused massage oils, creams, bath oils, and personal lubricants—especially women past menopause who suffer from dry vaginal membranes.

Pregnancy, Childbirth, and Recovery

Hemp has been there for women in their most vulnerable periods of life, acting as girlfriend, midwife, and doula, since the dawn of our relationship with herbs. She can help with menstrual irregularities, fertility, conception, and implantation. She relieves morning sickness, hyperemesis, anxiety, and insomnia. She relieves labor pain and can stimulate an arrested labor and elevate everyone in the birthing room to a spiritual place. She can relieve the pain of recovery and ensure a strong healthy child with a close bond to mother.

Concerns about safety for mother and child cannot be adequately addressed with modern research methods or surveys because they are stymied by politics and the illegal status of the herb. There have been some flawed and inconclusive experiments on mice and rats, and there have been a few surveys. Most of the surveys failed to separate out concomitant alcohol, tobacco, and other drug use during the pregnancy. (Not to mention environmental toxins.) Surveys also depend on mothers being brave enough to divulge their use of pot, when that admission comes with a high risk of stigma and severe legal sanctions that can lead to their children being taken from them or prison time or both. Surveys that did take these factors into account, like a 2002 survey of 12,060 British women, reported that marijuana has no reliable impact on birth size, physical abnormalities, length of gestation, or growth of the infant.[1]

However, from research into the ECS's role in the female reproductive system, from research into ancient use, and from modern stories of mothers and doctors, we can make good decisions concerning the use of cannabis during pregnancy, birth, and breastfeeding.[2]

The ECS is involved in the entire journey of pregnancy, starting with the health of the uterus and ovaries to the birth of a child and breastfeeding. Levels of endocannabinoids in a women's system regulate implantation, embryo development, and labor. Deficiencies in ECS function can lead to ectopic pregnancies, morning sickness, hyperemesis (severe nausea, vomiting, and weight loss), arrested labor, and even miscarriage. This suggests a role for cannabis supplementation. Supplementing with cannabis before pregnancy can enhance fertility. During pregnancy cannabis can quell nausea, increase appetite, reduce stress, improve sleep, and prevent miscarriage. As a birth aid it can reduce pain and invigorate stymied contractions. After the birth it can help with postpartum depression, pain, sleep, and the anxiety that comes with motherhood.

Let's look at some interesting examples: In Israel archeologists found evidence of birthing mothers using pot in a fourth century tomb. One wrote: "The woman was carrying a full-term fetus. The traces of cannabis . . . had been burned in a glass found by her side and must have been inhaled."[3] Another author observed: "Discovery of cannabis in the stomach of a pregnant woman buried west of Jerusalem confirms its use as an anesthetic during childbirth in the fourth century AD, if not before."[4]

Neurologist Ethan Russo tells us that Arabic medical texts from the ninth century recommend cannabis as useful to prevent miscarriage and to preserve fetuses in their mothers' abdomens. He also notes that the first Chinese materia medica, *Pen T'sao Kang Mu,* compiled in 1596, cites hemp seeds as a remedy for postpartum difficulties and the juice of the root as a remedy for retained placenta and postpartum hemorrhage.[5]

According to Dr. Russo, cannabinoids have been shown to diminish neuropathic pain associated with endometriosis, and endocannabinoids have been shown to modulate apoptosis in endometriosis and adenomyosis. Cannabis also has great potential to treat dysmenorrhea, premature labor, hyperemesis, and aid in childbirth postpartum hemorrhage, toxemic seizures, and menopause, according to Russo, and he believes that cannabis extracts may represent an efficacious and safe treatment for a wide range of conditions in women that interfere with fertility, a healthy pregnancy, and childbirth.[6]

In my travels in Southern Africa, I found that in many tribes there, including the Swazi, Zulu, Ndebele, and Sotho, mothers smoke copious amounts of dagga during labor. When I asked them why, their various reasons included to be brave, not feel pain, ensure a good birth, and have a healthy child. The shamans there (sangomas, or inyangas), often female, say that it is often the only time a woman will use dagga in her life.

In China and Southeast Asia, the ancient practice of cannabis use for childbirth continues today. In Cambodia, mothers sip hemp tea extensively after giving birth for a sense of well-being, to produce sufficient milk, and to alleviate postpartum stiffness. In Vietnam, they use hemp seeds to turn a fetus to a normal position during labor and for a feeling of wellness after childbirth. In China, hemp seeds are used for promoting lactation, hastening delivery, relieving birth pain, disinhibiting urination and defecation during labor, and to treat uterine prolapse and pain after birth.[7]

In India bhang has always been a birth aid, and British physicians learned about it thanks to a brilliant Irish physician named O'Shaughnessy. After serving his commission as an assistant surgeon in the East India Company from around 1830 to 1844, as mentioned previously, O'Shaughnessy brought Indian hemp back to Britain for the Pharmaceutical Society and the Royal Botanical Gardens, along with his extensive research into the history of medical uses of cannabis by ayurvedic and Persian physicians in India and the Middle East.* Below is a report from Sir Alexander Christison, a doctor, as included in an article by Ethan Russo:[8]

Indian hemp appears to possess a remarkable power of increasing the force of uterine contraction during labour . . .

One woman, in her first confinement, had forty minims of the tincture of cannabis one hour before the birth of the child. The os uteri was then of the size of a shilling, the parts very tender, with induration around the os uteri. The pains quickly became very strong, so much so as to burst the membranes, and project the liquor amnii to some distance, and soon the head was born. The uterus subsequently contracted well.

Another, in her first confinement, had one drachm of the tincture, when the os uteri was rigid, and the size of a half-crown; from this the labour became very rapid.

Another, in her first confinement, had also one drachm of the tincture, when the os uteri was the size of a half-crown. Labour advanced very rapidly, and the child was born in an hour and a-half. There were severe after-pains.

---

*He is also the doctor that the journal O'Shaughnessy's: The Journal of Cannabis in Clinical Practice is named for.

In 1851, Christison followed up his observations by saying:

> There appears little doubt, then, that the Indian hemp may often prove of essential service in promoting uterine contraction in tedious labours.[9]

Quite a few other British and Scottish physicians of that era noted that Indian hemp acted very quickly, often within minutes, to stimulate contractions in "tedious" births, reduced pain, and caused no unpleasant consequences in the mother nor abnormalities in the child. They noted that tinctures or concentrated extracts of Indian hemp made for a more pleasurable birth and a relaxed mother who recovered quickly. They also noted that when their pregnant patients were vomiting to an extent that threatened death, the vomiting completely ceased with cannabis indica.

One nineteenth-century Oxford professor, Philip Robson, summed it up well: "If you could have an agent which both speeded labour up, prevented hemorrhage after labour and reduced pain, this would be very desirable. Cannabis is so disreputable that nobody would begin to think of that and yet that is really an obvious application that we should seriously consider with perhaps some basic research and pursue it."[10]

A popular twentieth-century English text, *A Modern Herbal* by Maude Grieve, notes that "the [hemp] tincture helps parturition . . . An infusion of the seed is useful in after pains and prolapsus uteri."[11]

By far the best and most comprehensive research on the effects of ganja on mothers-to-be and children was done in the 1980s by nurse and anthropologist Melanie Dreher. To learn how prenatal marijuana use affected the neurobehavior of neonates and children, she chose to move from Columbia University to Jamaica to live with a very poor Jamaican community for two years. Jamaica's Rastafarian culture is wholly committed to ganja, and women there did not use alcohol, tobacco, or other drugs (see the Jamaica section in chapter 10). She compared thirty non-users of ganja with thirty ganja-using women there. Among the latter she witnessed a range of uses, including smoking, but most women sipped ganja tea and gave the tea to their children. They drank ganja to increase their appetites, prevent and control nausea, sleep better, and to give them the energy to work. They also reported that ganja helped them with the depression and desperation that attend motherhood in their impoverished communities. By drinking ganja tea, they could also prevent and improve colic in their infants and help them through teething.

At one-day-old and three-days-old, the two sets of infants showed no significant difference. At thirty-days-old, standardized neurobehavioral assessments showed that the "ganja babies" had better physiological stability, autonomic stability, quality of alertness, self-regulation, and less irritability. They thrived more and bonded better than the infants that were not exposed to marijuana in utero or through breast milk. In short, ganja use during pregnancy produced more robust babies.

Dreher was also able to do a five-year follow up to see how the children in her study were doing in school and at home. She asked their (educated, middle-class) teachers which children they thought received ganja tea at home. The teachers were shocked to learn that children from "ganja families" were the better dressed, better cared for, and more attentive students. No deleterious effects were ever noted from birth through age five.[12]

But what about in the United States? From 1971–1980, over two thousand children were delivered by midwives at the Farm, a community in Tennessee devoted to natural childbirth and midwifery. (By 2019, there had been over four thousand deliveries.) Expectant mothers came from all over the country to deliver their infants naturally. According to Dr. Jeffrey Hergenrather, the overseeing physician, about two-thirds of those mothers were using marijuana during their pregnancy. The infants were born healthy with no significant issues or negative scores in developmental tests. Ninety-five percent of the births occurred onsite, with only 5 percent being transferred to the local hospital. The need for cesarean sections was less than 2 percent, much lower than the national 25 percent rate.

Dr. Hergenrather participated in just four hundred of these births, as he was only called in when there was a difficulty that required an M.D. At those times, he saw marijuana used successfully and frequently during the birth process. "Often there would be a delay in labor, and I would be called in. Pot helped the delivery resume. It was fear that was causing the arrested labor. There was often an unresolved issue between the mother and father. After a joint was brought in and they both had a smoke, the couple would resolve the conflict, become all lovey-dovey, and labor would resume. I saw this over and over again."[13]

To sum up several medical professionals' perspective on using pot during pregnancy, I'll quote the Society of Cannabis Clinicians website: "After thoroughly discussing the risks and benefits with the mother, physicians should consider whether the patient's health is suffering more by not intaking cannabinoids during pregnancy."[14]

Dr. Wei-Ni Lin Curry has published her personal story of cannabis and hyperemesis gravidarum, a form of vomiting during pregnancy that goes way beyond morning sickness and can threaten the life of the fetus.

> Within two weeks of my daughter's conception, I became desperately nauseated and vomited throughout the day and night. . . . I vomited bile of every shade, and soon began retching up blood. . . . I felt so helpless and distraught that I went to the abortion clinic twice, but both times I left without going through with the procedure. . . . Finally, I decided to try medical cannabis. . . . Just one to two little puffs at night, and if I needed in the morning, resulted in an entire day of wellness. I went from not eating, not drinking, not functioning, and continually vomiting and bleeding from two orifices to being completely cured. . . . Not only did the cannabis save my [life] during the duration of my hyperemesis, it saved the life of the child within my womb."[15]

For decades Dr. Curry has lived where I do, in Northern California's Emerald Triangle, which has produced high-quality marijuana for the rest of the country since the early 1970s. There is less stigma here for pregnant women and mothers who use pot, and I have interviewed countless women about their use of cannabis during pregnancy, childbirth, and breastfeeding. I have never heard of any negative outcomes from this practice or had any mother say she regretted using marijuana in this way or felt that it had a negative impact on her child. I have heard many stories of how it helped, including the two below.

Kristi Edwards, a chiropractor in Northern California, told me:

> I was smoke-free until month five. But I was sooooooo nauseous all the time. The smell of food made me gag, all day, every day. I was exhausted. I lost twenty pounds my first four months. I kept waiting for the second trimester to feel better, but it never happened. So, I started smoking in the morning. It made a huge difference. Being able to eat brought my energy level up, and of course nourished baby D. I didn't smoke a lot, but it sure made me healthier.

Felicity's story is more detailed. She had happily smoked pot since she was a teenager. She worked on a community farm and had just picked up a trimming job at a marijuana farm when she realized she was pregnant and immediately cut back on her smoking to a couple of puffs every few days. She told me, "It was difficult because I was tired and nauseous all the time, so I wanted to smoke more . . . I felt like I was denying an instinct." But she was receiving a lot of negative judgment from her mother, who was convinced it would hurt the baby. The nausea reduced a bit during her second trimester, but she still felt lousy all the time—and guilty about the minimal amount she was smoking.

One beautiful spring day, she found herself farming barefoot in the sun and consciously decided to smoke a joint. "I instantly felt really connected to my body and my baby. I could actually see the baby inside of me. I dreamed of him that night. I know it, because when he was born, he looked exactly like my vision and my dream."

Felicity was in labor for almost four days in her birth hut. "By the third day, I got violently angry. The midwife had told me that I was dilated, and the contractions were still very intense. But my water hadn't broken yet, and then my cervix closed back up! I was throwing up so much that I passed out. We all decided to go to the hospital, where I received IV fluids and a Pitocin drip."

Although in a posterior position and resting on one of her nerves, which prevented her from moving or shifting position, her son was finally born after about seventy-five hours of labor. "I should have smoked during labor; it would have made me much more relaxed and might have shortened the time," Felicity realized. She returned to smoking regularly after the birth while raising her robust son on the farm.

Pregnant again three years later, she continued smoking throughout the pregnancy. She had separated from her abusive partner and noted, "Pot only helped the nausea a little, but it helped the stress a lot! I smoked after vomiting each time (several times a day) and I felt soooo much better afterward. I was older and more self-confident in following my instincts this time."

She developed symphysis pubis dysfunction (pelvic girdle pain and inflammation due to stiffening joints) with this pregnancy, which "made walking and just about everything hurt so so bad. . . It felt as if my pelvis was collapsing in on itself."

Felicity also had a fierce case of sciatica and two hernias, one umbilical and one in her groin. These caused excruciating pain, and she was hospitalized twice after episodes of vomiting and loss of consciousness.

With a daily ritual of smoking, applying salve frequently, and stretching, Felicity was able to care for her toddler and herself through the rest of her pregnancy. Here's how she described the birth:

Friends had given me a "birth joint" to use during labor this time. But I never had a chance. My daughter was born in a matter of minutes, while I was (thankfully) alone in the bedroom. I squatted and out she came. I caught her myself before anyone in the house knew what was happening. My water never broke this time either, but there was no pain at all and it was the most blissful experience I had ever had. It was actually orgasmic! For the next two weeks, the combination of marijuana and hormones kept me in that blissful state. My daughter came into the world healthy and bright-eyed. She gained weight rapidly. There were no issues whatsoever. I continue to smoke now while breastfeeding. I am a happy little clam . . . and so is she!

The Muscular System

Stiff, aching, and cramping muscles can quickly find relief with marijuana. For people with multiple sclerosis (2.5 million people worldwide) or spinal cord injury (15 million) who suffer from muscle spasticity, this can be a life-changing medicine, with none of the harmful side effects of prescription muscle relaxants. Of course, almost everyone experiences muscle tightness and cramping at some point in their lives. Topical use, internal use, and, my favorite, hot baths with cannabis leaves or cannabis-infused oil offer relief in most cases. Whether it is an athlete recovering from a workout, an elder experiencing nightly leg cramping or restless legs, or a woman experiencing uterine cramps, weed can save the day.

The Skeletal System

No bones about it, pot regulates and strengthens the skeletal system. Cannabis downregulates, or inhibits, the formation of osteoclasts, the cells that break down bone. This allows osteoblasts, cells that build bone, to catch up, especially in cases of osteoporosis and broken bones. As with the entire body, cannabis kills cancer cells in your bones (we will discuss this further in the "Cancer" section of this chapter).

The Gastrointestinal (GI) System

Within the gut, cannabis acts as an anti-inflammatory, helping with cases of colitis, pancreatitis, hepatitis, and diverticulosis. As an antispasmodic, cannabis reduces cramping and regulates the peristaltic contractions necessary to move your food through your tube. She nourishes and corrects imbalance in your enteric (GI) nervous system. Cannabis restores proper GI motility (uptake of nutrients), and her seeds and oil aid in overcoming constipation. She will patch leaky guts, rebalance diabetic conditions, and soothe an irritated bowel. She will kill intestinal parasites, and possibly prevent them. She can also tantalize the appetites of anorexics and AIDS patients. As with the entire body, in the GI tract cannabis kills cancer cells.

The Immune System

Outside of our brain, the greatest concentration of cannabinoid receptors is in our immune system. Many are located on our B lymphocytes, white blood cells that help produce immunoglobulins and antibodies. Cannabis is helpful not only in boosting our immunity but also in correcting autoimmune dysfunction diseases such as celiac disease, diabetes mellitus type 1, Graves' disease, inflammatory bowel disease, multiple sclerosis, psoriasis, rheumatoid arthritis, systemic lupus, Crohn's disease, and others. As in the whole body, she will kill cancer cells in the lymph system.

The Respiratory System

In the respiratory system, cannabis is anti-inflammatory and expectorant and slows and deepens breathing. Her essential oils are antiviral, antiseptic, calming, and inspiring. For those addicted to cigarettes, she will prevent lung cancer, throat cancer, and mouth cancer. For some, she will become a substitute for toxic cigarettes and help heal the addiction. We have even seen her reverse many of the symptoms of chronic obstructive pulmonary disease (COPD). As in the whole body, she will kill cancer cells in the respiratory system.

Jerry's Story

Jerry is a seventy-six-year-old retired engineer and avid cyclist. He came to me in 2016 searching for a good night's sleep. Averaging a mere four hours a night, he was waking in the early morning hours and was unable to go back to sleep. He had tried all the over-the-counter sleep aids. Although some provided a degree of help, he didn't like the harmful side effects and was now seeking nonharmful alternatives. Secondary issues for Jerry were asthma, high blood pressure (132/78 average), and restless leg syndrome.

We discussed his options and he decided to try Sleep Drops, a formula made with THCA-rich and CBD-rich cannabis as well as other common herbal sedatives. He started sleeping longer, although not all night, but enough to "help considerably."

During his second visit he wanted to address his lifelong dance with asthma. When he began developing an increased dependence on his albuterol inhaler in 1996, his doctor prescribed a corticosteroid inhaler called Asmanex and he decided to give it a try. He began using a 4,400 microgram (mcg) dose twice a day. It worked, and he was able to discontinue using the albuterol. Weekly air flow tests showed an average of about 280 liters/minute (400 l/m is the optimum range for someone of his age). Although extremely expensive, he was still using the same dosage with the same results twenty years later.

One aspect of asthma is chronic inflammation of the bronchial airways. Steroids help manage the symptoms because they are extremely anti-inflammatory—but they also carry harmful side effects. We began to explore other options and discussed the anti-inflammatory powers of cannabis and other herbs. Gary chose to try three different medicines. One was an anti-inflammatory alcohol tincture that contained THCA-rich cannabis and CBD-rich cannabis, formulated with other herbs. He also wanted to try a CBD-rich concentrate and some CBD-rich flower.

In January 2017 he began a cannabis therapy plan with the goal of eliminating his need for the corticosteroids. Initially he started with fifteen drops twice a day of the tincture and a large drop of the concentrate every other day in his food, while continuing to use the Asmanex. Here's how he described the effects: "After the first week on this regimen, my air flow increased [from 280 l/m] to an average of 335. The most obvious indication that things were different was that while riding in colder temperatures (40s) I no longer had the tightening in my bronchial tubes, which had been caused by the cold air rushing into my lungs. I mean, that was great—no tightness while climbing the hills!"

Jerry continued the same dosages for a total of three weeks, and his air flow increased to 370–390 l/m. "For an asthmatic," he said, "that is a huge increase! It gave me the confidence to reduce my dose of steroids by 25 percent from 880 to 660 mcg a day. Then during the fourth week, I started vaporizing CBD-rich cannabis. Initially, coughing was the reward, but I got the hang of it after a few days and settled on a regimen of two puffs twice a day (about 4 mg)."

By the fifth week, Jerry's air flow had increased to an average of 430 l/m with a high of 470. He was thrilled. In week six he reduced his Asmanex dose to 440 mcg, or half of the original dose. He also ran out of the CBD concentrate that week and replaced it with a similar one that also contained a high amount of THCA. His air flow dropped a little to average 410, but he was very happy with that. By the ninth week, Gary was using a total of 10 mg per day of CBD-rich, THCA-rich cannabis medicine. He continued to phase out the Asmanex, and his flow readings continued to be in the 410 range. By the tenth week, he discontinued the Asmanex altogether. Jerry reports:

"I'm happy. Now, a year later, my flow meter readings remain in the 400s. I have reduced my cannabinoid dosage to about 7 mg per day, and vaporize about three times a week, for a total of 9 mg of CBD-rich cannabinoids. I do notice when using the vaporizer that my air flow will increase after about five minutes. I took some of Wendy's classes, and now I grow my own CBD-rich cannabis and make my own oil-based tinctures. In my case, asthma is caused by inflammation, irritants, allergies, and emotional stress. It cannot be cured. Through my use of CBD-rich cannabis, I have been able to control inflammation and reduce emotional stress and anxiety. Regarding environmental aspects, maybe my tolerance levels have even increased, I don't know.

Other unexpected but positive results of my cannabis therapy plan are that my blood pressure is now down to an average of 112/68, my glucose levels are down from 108 to 96, and my restless legs are no longer restless! Oh, and the side effects of corticosteroids? Gone!"

By 2019 his cannabis therapy had brought Jerry back into balance. He ceased using his vaporizer on a regular basis and now only needs it when environmental issues such as smoke causes tightness in his chest. He continues to use a maintenance dose of 10 mg of CBD-rich cannabis tincture a day.

The Cardiovascular System

Cannabis is an adaptogen, an herb that helps your body adapt to stress physically, mentally, and spiritually. In your cardiovascular system, marijuana will tone blood vessels, correct blood pressure, and remove and prevent plaque buildup in the arteries. She will give you the antioxidant strength needed to protect you from tissue damage during a stroke or a heart attack. Her stress-relieving abilities will prevent strokes, panic attacks, and heart attacks. One molecule (THC) in whole plant cannabis will increase your heart rate and strengthen your heartbeat. A different molecule in the plant (CBD) will do the opposite. Presented together with the rest of their plant team, they will bring your cardiovascular system back into homeostasis. As in the whole body, she will kill cancer cells in the blood.

The Nervous System

Cannabis is the queen of nervines, herbs that support and heal the nervous system, and the other neurotransmitters are her handmaidens, rushing through the palace corridors to do her bidding. She will clothe naked nerves in a healthy myelin sheath, keep suicidal thoughts at bay while she rebalances your brain chemistry, and order the growth of new healthy nerves at the same time she eases the pain of the dying ones. She can quell your anxiety and she will help you sleep. In many cases she can quell seizures, tremors, and convulsions. As in the whole body, she will kill cancer cells in the brain and nervous system.

Skin

Our skin is our largest organ and our primary defense from microbes and illness. Dry skin is compromised skin, so we must keep hydrated with both water and oils for the skin to be a healthy barrier. Healthy skin is an important component in hair growth and our ability to sweat and release toxins. Cutaneous endocannabinoids maintain skin homeostasis and regeneration.

Common skin ailments, like dermatitis (inflammation), psoriasis (autoimmune disorder), acne, eczema, and cancers may indicate a deficiency in the ECS. They can often be successfully treated with topically applied cannabis medicine, as well as internal use. (See Rick Simpson's story in chapter 6.)

Sleep

Insomnia is a holistic and complex condition. Everyone's insomnia is different and usually requires a personal consultation to narrow down what is going on. Because cannabis is biphasic and can have different and sometimes opposing effects depending on the dosage, a low dose of THC can be stimulating and a high dose sedating. This also means that what is a sedative dose for one person can be stimulating to another. (There is more about this in the anxiety section of chapter 4.) Herbal sedatives can have an affinity for calming the mind or the body, and I make different recipes for each. In cases of challenged sleep, I prefer tinctures to teas, as they can be kept next to the bed and don't make you have to get up to pee. Both of my remedies have low doses of low-THC cannabis. If that doesn't work for a client, I consider recommending that they carefully try a high dose of THC in an edible or concentrated medicine.

DISEASES OF THE BODY

Cancer

Every day, thousands of people around the world cure their cancers by using natural medicine. No one in the United States is recording or reporting on this, and many doctors and clinics here that have successfully healed cancers naturally have been pressured to leave the country by the American Medical Association and the government. So, most Americans believe that big pharma is their only remedy of choice.

Many cancer patients come to me after completing the allopathic treatment plan of surgery, chemotherapy, and radiation because it didn't work for them. Since everyone's cancer holds a different place in their minds, bodies, and spirits, how can a treatment plan—especially one that consists solely of allopathic medicine—be one-size-fits-all? Yet hundreds of thousands of people with breast cancer, for example, receive the same surgery, chemotherapy, and radiation. And after all of that medical care, why can they still not answer this question: What should *I* do to heal my cancer? Let's explore more deeply to see if we can understand not just cancer but the cancer that is unique within all of us.

Every day, your healthy cells experience mutations in their DNA, mostly from environmental pollution in the air, soil, food, and water. Corrective teams of molecules regularly go into your DNA and repair these mutations. If your cells cannot be repaired, they are programmed to self-destruct, which prevents them from replicating along with their damaged DNA. This natural process is happening continually at a low level, and the body easily processes and eliminates these dead cells. This "cellular suicide" is called apoptosis.

If someone's immune system, or whole being, becomes overwhelmed and out of balance, these corrective measures cannot keep up. When mutations accumulate in the genes that control cell division and apoptosis, including tumor suppression genes, cancer erupts. Most cancer cells develop only after over sixty mutations! Then growth-promoting genes become hyperactive, causing the cells to divide uncontrollably. Because these cells are still part of the organism and are not an outside "invader" like a virus or bacteria, the immune system does not eliminate them. Cancer cells hide from your immune system.

As these cancer cells rapidly divide and begin to form growths, they design and develop their own vascular system—veins, arteries, capillaries—the whole shebang. This is called angiogenesis. Now called tumors, they can mine the blood for sugar and nutrients. The tumors then start secreting enzymes that break down and weaken the surrounding healthy tissues, thus allowing the cancer to expand into new territory. These enzymes, called proteases, can also break down the adhesive that holds the cells together, so cancerous cells can slip into the blood or lymph systems and travel to a new spot—a journey called metastasis.

Apoptosis is just one of the ways a cell can die; the other way is by necrosis, which is when a cell ruptures or explodes due to outside forces like blunt trauma or pharmaceutical drugs. When many sick cells explode like this, they leak too much poison into a system that is struggling to clean them up. For example, if a person who is struggling with Lyme disease and already has a compromised immune system uses large doses of antibiotics to kill Lyme disease bacteria, a toxic overload results and they often become sicker. This is called a Herxheimer, or a "Herx," reaction. The same thing happens with chemotherapy or radiation, which leads patients to feel worse and further overloads their already taxed immune systems.

Cannabis, and other herbs and foods, naturally induce apoptosis, and not necrosis. That is why they do not cause side effects and also boost the immune system rather than taxing it.

But how does cannabis kill cancer? In a 1975 American study, published in the *Journal of the National Cancer Institute,* researchers shared how cannabis prevents angiogenesis, the formation of blood vessels in tumors, and also dissolves any existing blood vessels in the tumor.[16] This is one way that she shrinks tumors—often down to nothing. Decades of studies have since demonstrated the anticancer activity of cannabis in dozens of different types of cancers in the breast, prostate, colon, skin, lung, and mouth as well as lymphomas.[17]

In 1998 researchers in Spain discovered that THC can induce apoptosis of cancer cells.[18] This means it selectively induces programmed cell death in those cells without negatively impacting surrounding healthy cells. As opposed to chemotherapy—which indiscriminately kills through necrosis any fast-growing cells in the body, including hair follicles and the cells in the stomach lining—pot reduces the toxic load on the immune system while killing cancer cells.

By 2004 even the *Journal for the American Association of Cancer Research* reported that cannabis inhibits the metastasis, or spread, of cancer, and the University of South Florida found that THC can inhibit the gamma herpes virus, a potential cause of Kaposi's sarcoma, Burkitt's lymphoma, and Hodgkin's disease.[19]

In 2007 Harvard researchers found that cannabis inhibits the growth of lung cancer. It was also found to stop the growth of glioblastoma brain cancer cells.[20]

In 2012 scientists in San Francisco found that THC stops metastasis.[21] One way it does so is by protecting the healthy cells around the cancer. Cannabis will also protect tissues and organs from environmental toxins; thus, it is a wonderful adjunct for those who chose toxic therapies like chemotherapy and radiation.

Cannabis boosts the immune system. Outside of the brain, the highest concentration of cannabinoid receptors is found in the immune system, specifically on the B lymphocytes. Cancer is "caused" by an overwhelmed immune system, and cannabis is an antidote.

Cannabis, specifically CBD, can turn off an active ID1 gene. This gene is active in fetal development when cells need to divide rapidly and differentiate into different kinds of cells, like heart cells, skin cells, etc. The ID1 gene normally turns off at birth, but in some cases of cancer, it turns back on again, causing uncontrolled, rapid cell division leading to tumors. Cannabis can turn off this gene.

The National Cancer Institute finally published the following statement in March of 2011:

> Cannabinoids may cause antitumor effects by various mechanisms, including induction of cell death, inhibition of cell growth and inhibition of tumor angiogenesis and metastasis. Cannabinoids appear to kill tumor cells but do not affect their non-transformed counterparts and may even protect them from cell death.
>
> . . . The potential benefits of medicinal cannabis for people living with cancer include antiemetic effects, appetite stimulation, pain relief and improved sleep. In the practice of integrative oncology, the health care provider may recommend medicinal cannabis not only for symptom management but also for its possible direct antitumor effect.[22]

Cannabis expert Dr. William Courtney shared a story on the Cure Your Own Cancer website about his youngest patient, eight months old, with a massive, centrally located, inoperable brain tumor. His parents put cannabis oil on the baby's pacifier twice a day, slowly increasing the dose. Within two months there was a dramatic reduction in the tumor. After eight months the tumor was much further reduced, and the family was able to avoid all the side effects and risks of chemotherapy and radiation.[23]

COVID

In the spring of 2020, for the first time in human history, the entire world was focused on the same thing: the SARS-CoV2 coronavirus (COVID). According to Wikipedia, by July 2022 an estimated 554 million people worldwide had been infected by COVID. At this point everyone is aware that the severity of the disease can range from asymptomatic carriers to "flu-like" cases that cause headaches, body aches, and chest congestion to cases so severe that they result in long-term—possibly permanent—illness, brain damage, or death.

Marijuana has over five hundred fifty medicinal chemicals and many of them are already known to be antiviral, including but not limited to cannabinoids, cannabinoid acids, and terpenes. They work together to protect the immune system from dysfunction. It's important to understand that cannabis medicine does not shut down the entire immune system like the currently used steroid therapy does, which leaves a patient vulnerable to all disease. Instead, it promotes a healthy immune response. Marijuana inhibits or blocks viral actions including attachment, spike protein formation, protease production, replication, and gene expression. Cannabis medicine helps the body keep or retain interferon function and prevents inflammatory cytokine storms. It protects healthy tissue from viral infection and its effects, including within the vascular endothelium and the brain. Marijuana acts as a bronchodilator, expectorant, analgesic, and anti-inflammatory, which means that during infection, it will help relieve the worst symptoms of COVID, including breathing difficulties, lung congestion, head and body aches, inflammation, nausea, vomiting, and diarrhea. Below we'll discuss recent in vitro (test tube) studies that give evidence of marijuana's anti-COVID properties.

The coronavirus uses spike proteins on its coat to penetrate host cells. The virus's favorite ports of entry are ACE2 receptors (angiotensin-converting enzyme 2), which are found throughout the mucous membranes of the lungs, mouth, nose, kidneys, testes, GI tract, and, most notably, in the brain and in the endothelium (inner lining) of our veins, arteries, and capillaries. Once it merges with a host cell, the virus stimulates the release of a protease enzyme (TMPRSS2) to weaken surrounding cell membranes, force entry, and hijack their DNA to begin replicating itself. Because the virus can spread cell-to-cell, thereby avoiding the antibodies cruising through the bloodstream, it can hide from the immune system.

Marijuana medicine prevents and treats COVID in a myriad of ways. Cannabis boosts the ECS to prevent viral attachment by inhibiting the formation of the viral spike proteins and protects surrounding healthy cells by inhibiting TMPRSS2.[24] CBD has been shown to expose hidden infected cells to the immune system and block viral replication in the epithelial cells lining the lungs and other implantation sites like oral and nasal passages.[25] It also inhibits viral gene expression. Cells treated with CBD retain this ability even after the virus is gone. Patients that are already using CBD regularly show a lower incidence of infection upon exposure.[26]

The essential oils of cannabis contain many anti-COVID terpenes, including beta-myrcene, alpha- and beta-pinene, limonene, beta-ocimene, and 1,8-cineole, that inhibit viral replication.[27] Regularly inhaling (huffing) these essential oils, or dotting them on your mask, scarf, or shirt can give you continuous protection. Alternatively, you can tuck a piece of an aromatic herb, like cannabis or lavender, into your mask. (I like peppermint because it also opens the sinus passageways.) Diluting an essential oil with olive oil, another carrier oil, or skin lotion, allows you to safely apply it directly on your skin. (Remember, undiluted essential oils can burn!) You can also suck on cough drops like Ricolas or candy like Altoids, as they contain essential oils. (The old Vicks VapoRub contains a lot of essential oils, but it has a poisonous petroleum base, so I do not recommend that.) Gargling cannabis tea or using it to clear nasal passages may significantly prevent, slow, or stop viral progress. Filling a room with smoke from an herbal incense or smudge, including pot, can clear it of bacterial and fungal pathogens for up to twenty-four hours.[28] I suspect it might kill viruses as well, but there has been no research in this area.

If the virus invades the stomach, causing nausea, vomiting, diarrhea, cramping or abdominal pain, consuming cannabis (tea, edibles, tinctures, or oils) will help these symptoms as well as prevent replication. If the patient can't keep anything down, they can smoke or vaporize for immediate, if not as long-lasting, relief.

One of the ways that COVID suppresses the immune system is by inhibiting interferon cytokines that signal the presence of infection and activate natural killer cells (T lymphocytes) and macrophages. CBD upregulates the interferon pathway, essentially returning its function.[29]

If the virus infects the inner lining of the vascular system, trouble abounds. The vascular endothelium plays a huge role in regulating immune function and inflammatory equilibrium by preventing blood clots, by keeping the vascular endothelial membranes toned and semipermeable, and by keeping blood flow stable. Viral disruption of these functions can cause major problems including blood clots, strokes, ischemic events, cytokine storms (systemic hyperinflammation), and severe dysfunction of immune cells including T lymphocytes, macrophages, interferon, and B lymphocytes (antibody producers), which all work together to clear viral infections.[30] Cannabis prevents viral attachment and replication in the vascular system and inhibits inflammatory cytokine storms.[31]

One of the fastest ways to get cannabis into your bloodstream, where it will protect the endothelial cells and prevent inflammation and clotting, is an alcohol tincture held under the tongue. Consuming edibles will also get it there, just not as quickly.

Inhaling cannabis—vaporized or even smoked—acts as an immediate bronchodilator, expectorant, and anti-inflammatory for congested lungs. It can also prevent the virus from attaching and replicating in the mouth, nose, throat, and lungs. That said, I do know many pot smokers that have gotten COVID, but without research, I don't know if their cases were less severe due to their cannabis use. Many of those with lung symptoms reported that smoking was the only thing that opened up their lungs and allowed them to cough up phlegm.

One of the scariest parts of COVID is its neurological effects. Several viruses, like the H1N1 virus (Spanish flu), Middle East respiratory syndrome (MERS), and severe acute respiratory syndrome (SARS), cause neurological symptoms including sleep disruption, extreme fatigue, moderate to severe headaches, drowsiness, coma, restlessness, and tremors.[32] COVID not only causes a significant increase in the frequency and severity of these symptoms, it brings with it additional, more severe problems like delirium, altered taste and smell, and long-lasting/permanent neurological and psychiatric conditions, including strokes, brain hemorrhaging, brain damage, memory loss, inability to concentrate, psychosis, seizures, and Alzheimer's disease.

One study reviewed over 236,000 COVID cases for six months following hospitalization and found that 84 percent of COVID patients had at least one first-ever diagnosis of a neurological or psychiatric disorder, including nerve disorders, strokes, dementia myoneural disease, psychosis, and brain hemorrhage among others. The study also found that neurological and psychiatric problems occur at a high rate in light-to-moderate cases that did not require hospitalization.[33]

With COVID, neurological infections often appear before the first onset of respiratory symptoms and are sometimes the only presenting symptoms. More than half of hospitalized COVID patients experience encephalopathy (altered brain function or structure), which leads to a higher incidence of strokes and seizures. One study found an average of twelve days of acute brain dysfunction, including comas.[34] Other studies show that over 90 percent of hospitalized COVID patients have reported at least one neurological effect that continued six months after hospitalization, and long-term brain damage has occurred in as many as one quarter of COVID survivors regardless of the severity of the initial disease.[35]

These cognitive impairments are not due to hypoxia (lack of oxygen to the brain caused by breathing difficulties) but by a viral invasion of the brain. When the virus is inhaled, the body sends in immune cells that release inflammatory cytokines that change the olfactory nerve cells and prevent odor receptors from functioning, even though the virus doesn't infect the neurons themselves. These neurons are connected to areas of the brain that influence cognition and emotions. The spike proteins on the viral coat allow the virus to break through the blood-brain barrier and head to the hippocampus. Since the brain does not have an immune response, the virus likes to hide there, freely replicating or going dormant only to reactivate at a later date.

Postmortem analyses have shown brains that contained one thousand times higher levels of the virus than other parts of the body.[36] Inflammation in the brain ensues as the virus uses brain cells to replicate and also kills surrounding healthy neurons by changing the brain's vasculature to deprive the cells of oxygen. These ischemic infarctions create permanent brain damage—and, like in other parts of the body, long-term low-level inflammation in the brain can lead to autoimmune disease in the CNS.[37] Other studies report loss of gray matter, brain volume, atrophy in the cerebellum, tissue damage in the olfactory cortex, and increases in cerebrospinal fluid.[38]

Patients with brain damage are at a high risk of developing neurodegenerative diseases, like Parkinson's and multiple sclerosis, or general cognitive decline. The virus can also cause tau proteins to build up in the brain (due to dysfunctional ryanodine receptors), which are associated with Alzheimer's disease and dementia: 66 percent of patients over age sixty-five, and 72 percent who had encephalopathy, receive a first diagnosis of dementia within six months of having COVID.[39]

Cannabis crosses the blood-brain barrier and can offer its antiviral, tissue-protectant, and anti-inflammatory medicine to the CNS in addition to preventing and treating twisted tau proteins. I have had several cases where habitual cannabis users had an altered sense of smell, but so far I've seen no permanent damage or long-COVID cases coming from that cohort.

Although science picks her apart in their studies, remember that whole plant cannabis medicine is her most powerful form. In addition to her antiviral and protective qualities, marijuana provides additional support to patients by helping with any depression, anxiety, or boredom that often comes with severe or long-term illness. Lastly, but maybe most importantly, she provides spiritual connection and support during life-changing, or deadly, illness.

General Symptoms That Cannabis Can Relieve

Symptoms of ADD and ADHD

Addiction

Anxiety

Constipation

Convulsions

Depression

Diarrhea

Inflammation: Including but not limited to the lungs (bronchitis, asthma), the gut (colitis, Crohn's disease), the brain (Alzheimer's disease, dementia), the muscular/skeletal system (osteoarthritis, rheumatoid arthritis), the uterus, systemic inflammation (lupus), and inflammation caused by or affected by cancer

High cholesterol

High or low blood pressure

Inability to focus on or pay attention to one thing at a time

Insomnia

Lack of appetite

Leaky gut

Morning sickness

Muscle spasms

Nausea, vomiting

Pain: Including but not limited to neuropathic pain, migraines, menstrual pain, cancer pain, and arthritis

Racing thoughts or circular thinking

Seizures

Stress symptoms

Symptoms of metabolic disorders: Including but not limited to diabetes and obesity

Tinnitus

Weak or broken bones

6

Types of Marijuana Medicine

Because of our co-creative relationship with cannabis, humans can ingest her in myriad ways. You have ancestors somewhere in your lineage who used this herb simply, safely, and effectively—otherwise you wouldn't be here! Your ancestors used this magical plant in all its forms in the kitchen, operating room, sauna, bedroom, and most everywhere else. People have been eating her, smoking her, drinking infusions, and rubbing her on our skin for millennia. This plant really wants to be inside of us—so badly that she will enter through our nose, mouth, ears, skin, eyes, rectum, vagina, and consciousness. We can inhale her scent in the garden or as steam, incense, smoke, or vapor. We can sip her as tea, or in coffee, cocoa, milk, beer, wine, or cocktails. We can eat her in any recipe or on her own. We can bathe in her and pack our wounds with her. We can dose ourselves with her via flower essences, tinctures, vinegars, oils, or concentrates. Each of these methods is beneficial, and each has its advantages. For much more on the ancient uses of cannabis, see chapter 10. There are detailed instructions about how to make many marijuana medicines in chapter 9. Here we will describe the myriad of medicines that you can choose from.

With herbs, there is no such thing as a dose that suits all people or animals, or a medicine that suits a certain disease or illness. There are only dosages and medicines that suit individuals, and they can change all the time. New users of cannabis therapy should start low and go slow;

avoid THC edibles until you determine your sensitivity using another, milder method of ingestion; and continually evaluate the effects of your plan and make adjustments as necessary. Above all, don't be afraid to just try a small dose of whichever THC medicine you are attracted to.

There are five things to consider when choosing medicines for yourself or a client: time of onset of the effect, duration of the effect, risk of THC overdose, target areas, and conditions that the medication is ideal for. Each of these five considerations are explored for each type of medicine covered in the following pages.

TOPICALS

Applying hemp to the skin is an ancient tradition in many cultures. Topically applied medicines include concentrates, liniments, infused oils, salves, lotions, skin creams, hydrosols, essential oils, personal lubricants, sitz baths, poultices, compresses, and bath bags. THC topical medicines are not psychoactivating, yet they can be very spirit-activating!

Time of onset: Immediate to 20 minutes
Duration of effect: 1–6 hours
Risk of THC overdose: Zero
Target areas: Skin, joints, muscles
Conditions topicals are ideal for: Joint, muscle, and neuropathic pain; inflammation; burns; muscle spasms; wounds; broken bones; skin and blood infections including MRSA; skin cancer and cancers that are just under the skin, like melanoma, prostate, breast, or thyroid cancer.

Liniments
When applied topically, alcohol tinctures are called liniments. They can carry medicine through the skin and into the muscles, joints, and bloodstream. Eighteenth- and nineteenth-century physicians and veterinarians relied heavily on alcohol extracts, and the American and European pharmacopoeias are full of cannabis tinctures and liniments.

Poultices

A poultice is a topical application of prepared plant matter. Hemp poultices have been used around the world in many cultures for thousands of years. The herbs can be dried and powdered, fresh and well-pounded, chewed up, or briefly boiled in water. Alcohol can be added to increase absorption. Poultices can be packed directly onto wounds, burns, bruises, cuts, scrapes, rashes, hemorrhoids, infections, skin cancers, and other skin conditions. They are good for postpartum bleeding, gout, inflammation, muscle injuries and spasms, broken bones, lung infections, and tumors and growths. Often when you remove them, they have absorbed the toxins or infection from the wound and turned dark or slimy. You can tell they are doing their job! They are non-psychoactive.

Infused Oils for Topical Use

Herbal oils, or infused oils, and the art of massage therapy both developed in arid regions where water was a scarce resource. In the deserts of the Middle East and in Africa and India where there was no water for bathing, people cleaned themselves and each other by rubbing oil into the skin. In place of soap, desert tribes infused their oils with herbs, both for their heady aromas and for their medicinal, hygienic, and spiritual qualities. (See The Hebrews section in chapter 10). Herb-infused oils are good for hair conditioning, skin conditioning, skin issues, massage, bruises, broken bones, arthritis and joint issues, chronic pain, inflammation, and sexual enhancement. Herbal oils are subtle, potent, valuable, and can be made at home by steeping dried or fresh herbs in vegetable oil with gentle heat for a period of time. (Not to be confused with essential oils, which are distilled.) Chemical constituents are "digested" from the herbs into the oil. Cannabinoid-containing trichome crystals are oil soluble, as are hemp's essential oils, flavonoids, and alkaloids. Infused oils are often used as the base for salves, skin creams, and lotions. When applied topically, cannabis-infused oils are non-psychoactive, but may be spiritually activating.

Warning: Pesticides are also soluble in oil.

Salves

Salves are topically applied ointments used to protect the skin and to apply herbal medicine. They are potent, portable, and can easily be made at home. Salves are typically a blend of oils and solid fats like cocoa butter or beeswax. Lip balms and ChapStick are salves, as is Tiger Balm. Cannabis salves are excellent for skin conditions including cancer, burns, bruises, eczema, and psoriasis. They often provide immediate relief for pain and inflammation of the spine and joints. They are nonpsychoactive.

> **Warning:** Commercial salves are often petroleum-based and therefore poisonous. They may contain pesticides and other toxins.

Bert's Story

My friend Jan's sixty-year-old husband, Bert, suffered from knee pain ever since he played football in college. His left knee never fully recovered from a torn anterior cruciate ligament (ACL), and he compensated by overusing his right knee. By age thirty-eight, osteoarthritis had set into both knees. He experienced pain and inflammation regularly, and due to limited mobility had become obese with the threat of diabetes hovering over him. Now fifty years old, he needed one and perhaps two knee replacements, but since the life expectancy of a new knee was only twenty years he wanted to wait until he was at least fifty-five. When medical marijuana became legal in his state, he tried smoking a joint—something he had not done since college. Although it relaxed him and lifted his spirits, it did not help with the pain in his knees.

Jan called me asking for advice. "Has he tried a salve?" I asked. I explained the potential benefits, and she sent Bert to the new dispensary in town. Only at the third dispensary he tried did he find, way in a back corner, some small jars of a cannabis ointment. At home he applied it liberally to both knees, rubbing it in thoroughly for about *five minutes. Then he stood up to walk around the room. The pain in his right knee was completely gone. Even the pain in his left knee was now bearable! Shocked and elated, he went out the front door and proceeded to walk down his driveway, and then around the block—something he never would have considered before. The effect of the salve lasted about three hours until pain and inflammation returned. He iced both knees and reapplied the salve. It worked again!*

By applying the salve three or four times a day Bert could walk a mile around the local track. He began to lose a little weight, and this inspired him to clean up his diet to ward off diabetes. The store-bought salve was expensive, so Jan came to me to learn how to make her own. Her son was now growing marijuana in his backyard and gave her all the leaves and trim.

"I still plan to have my left knee replaced in a few years," Bert says, "but for now I have less pain and swelling than I've had my whole adult life. It truly is a miracle, this little salve, and now I give it away to my old football buddies all the time. They love it, too!"

Herbal Soaks

After a long day of work, what feels better than slipping your feet into a basin of hot water or your whole body into a hot tub infused with salts, herbs, and oils? Mental stress and anxiety can float away, and tired, aching muscles and joints get the relaxation and rejuvenation they deserve. The simple addition of Epsom salts will draw out any infections or toxins, and the body can absorb its magnesium through the skin to help with restless legs or muscle cramps. Many medicinal qualities of marijuana and other herbs can also be absorbed through soaking or bathing. After all, the bottoms of our feet are very porous and were designed to absorb medicine from the powerful but tiny weeds that we walk on.

Any part of a pot plant can be added to a soak, and so can infused oils or essential oils. Salves can be applied to specific areas before we dip in. For my clients I often make personalized herbal blends in giant tea bags for hand or foot soaks, baths, or steams. Soaks are good for anxiety, insomnia, meditation, joints, muscles, skin issues, and respiratory issues. Hydrotherapy, the alternation of hot and cold therapies, is extremely effective for poor circulation, stagnant lymph, chronic and acute joint issues, muscle spasms, restless legs, night cramps, and improved immune function. All soaks will increase circulation and interrupt the patterns of chronic inflammation. Non-psychoactive.

INGESTED MEDICINES

Fresh Weed

I love fresh green marijuana sprinkled on my salad or in my smoothies, salsas, and pestos. Even in sauerkraut! The medical benefits of fresh raw cannabis leaf and flower was first "re"-discovered by Emerald Triangle pot doc Dr. William Courtney. He recommended the fresh herb as a nutritious vegetable that should be regularly consumed like spinach and other dark green leafy vegetables. Not only is ganja leaf salad or juice nutritious, it also has anticancer and anti-inflammatory properties. And even the stoniest pot can be consumed fresh and remain non-psychoactive.

Since fresh cannabis is not always available, we often preserve it by freezing it, tincturing it, or juicing it and preserving the juice with alcohol (a succuss), sugar or honey (a syrup), or in the freezer.

Tea Time

When someone comes to me upset or just wanting to talk, one of the first things I do is to start a pot of tea. This has the immediate effect of reassuring them that they are welcome and that I want to take the time to listen. Herbal tea is a gentle way to introduce someone to marijuana. Many of my elder clients love the tea blends I make for them, and they are easy to slip into their routines. Children love tea, especially when sweetened with a bit of stevia or honey. Tea is a relaxing ritual. After incense, teas are one of the oldest ways that humans have communed with ganja. (See the sections about bhang in chapter 10.)

Like all herbs, weed works better when combined with other herbs, so you can brew a cup with just ganja or include some pot leaves in your favorite tea blend.

Time of onset: Slower than inhaling, faster than edibles .
Duration of effect: 1–3 hours
Risk of THC overdose: Depends on preparation, see below
Target areas: Digestive tract, nervous system, internal organs, spiritual communion
Conditions tea is ideal for: Most conditions

🌿 Fresh Cannabis Sun Tea

Add 1–3 grams of fresh cannabis leaves or flowers per cup of room temperature water in a glass container with a lid. Feel free to add some of your favorite tea herbs and some more water for medicine or flavor. Leave covered outside in the sun for an hour. Filter and serve at room temperature or iced. Non-psychoactive.

🌿 Dried Cannabis Sun Tea

Add 1 gram of dried leaf or flower per cup of room temperature water in a glass container with a lid. Feel free to add some of your favorite tea herbs and some more water for medicine or flavor. Leave covered outside in the sun for an hour. Filter and serve at room temperature or iced. Very low psychoactivity.

🌿 Hot Teas

Add 1 gram of dried leaf or 3 grams of fresh leaf per cup of hot water. Feel free to add some of your favorite tea herbs and some more water for medicine or flavor. Add some hemp milk, hemp seed milk, whole milk, ghee, or coconut oil. Steep covered for 5 minutes. Filter and serve hot or cold. Gently psychoactive to psychoactive.

Inhalants

Although given a bad rap over the years and mistakenly labeled "bad for you," smoking pot is actually good for you on many levels! There are many advantages to inhaling your marijuana medicine, and there are many ways to do it. Smoking or vaporizing leaf or flower is one of the best and fastest ways to determine initial dosages. You can start with a small inhalation and immediately feel if it is enough. You can quickly take a second "hit" if one is not enough, and repeat until you feel a desired effect. From there, you can determine initial doses for other methods of ingestion, like edibles or tinctures.

Time of onset: Immediate

Duration of effect: Short. The full effect of inhalation spikes quickly, then falls away within half an hour to an hour. This is reassuring in those rare cases where the effect is unpleasant for someone. It is a disadvantage for those who want a longer-lasting effect, like sleeping through the night, being out of pain, or for chronic inflammation.

Risk of THC overdose: Very low

Target areas: Mouth, sinuses, trachea, lungs, brain (from the lungs, the blood flow carries it directly to the brain)

Conditions inhalation is ideal for: Pain, appetite stimulation, spiritual communion, relationships, emotional state, cancer, and other diseases in target areas. Reduces risk of lung disease in cigarette smokers.

Vaporizing

Vaporizing the cannabis crystals off the buds is a popular way to take in her terpenes and cannabinoids. Little to no combustion of plant material (smoke) is involved. People also vaporize concentrated cannabis oils, like high critical CO_2 extractions or those made with other, more toxic solvents like dabs or shatter. The safest way to vape is by using buds or leaves in a volcano-style vaporizer, because there are no other chemicals involved. As explained in more detail in the concentrates section of this chapter, be wary of vape pens that contain metal wires to heat the medicine as you will be slowly inhaling the metal wire too. Also avoid cartridges of concentrated oils that contain any toxic chemicals like artificial flavors or propylene glycol. Vaporizing THCA or THC is psychoactive.

Smoking

Smoking marijuana is not bad for your lungs! In fact, it helps prevent lung cancer if you also smoke cigarettes.[1] It does not cause COPD or other lung diseases. Marijuana smoke is tissue protective and a bronchodilator and expectorant; for some, it relieves asthma. However, everyone is different, and if you find that smoking irritates your lungs or throat, try another method of ingestion. Avoid lighting anything you smoke with butane lighters, as you will also be inhaling the butane, which is toxic and a throat irritant. Use matches or, even better, a magnifying glass in the sun to take "solar hits." Smoking THCA or THC plants or medicines is psychoactive.

Aerosols

Spraying and inhaling hydrosols or diluted essential oils is another way to calm lung spasms, kill respiratory pathogens, and calm or prevent anxiety attacks. Spraying wounds prevents and treats infection and inflammation. Spritzers cool the skin and perk you up. Non-psychoactive.

Steams

Steam inhalation of essential oils or inhaling the steam from a hot cannabis tea is a very gentle way to get medicine to the lungs. Long before there were pharmaceutical inhalers, steam inhalation of eucalyptus and peppermint were the only treatments for asthma. Now we can add the wonderful anti-inflammatory, antimicrobial, anticancer, and bronchodilating effects of cannabis, too. Non-psychoactive.

Tinctures and Sublingual Sprays

Tinctures are a great choice for mimicking our own endocannabinoids and restoring balance to our system. They also excel at boosting the immune system. They are a gentle introduction to the oral consumption of THC.

Once our ancestors discovered the art of distillation, they began using spirits to infuse and preserve their herbs. We call these tinctures. Usually they are made with alcohol. Tinctures with over 40 percent (80 proof) alcohol have an indefinite lifespan. Alcohol will preserve cannabinoid acids, like THCA or CBDA, indefinitely, preventing them from breaking down into their neutral cannabinoids like THC or CBD. Alcohol carries medicine into your bloodstream very rapidly, as it can be absorbed directly through the skin or the mucous membranes of your mouth before you even swallow. Tinctures can be psychoactive if they contain decarboxylated THC. Many tinctures are made without heat and are therefore non-psychoactive because the THC is present in its non-psychoactive THCA form. When taken orally, within minutes the medicine absorbs into the blood system from the mouth, and very little travels into the rest of the digestive system unless there is something edible in it, like glycerin or honey.

Glycerin has weaker extracting and preserving abilities than alcohol, but makes a nice substitute for recovering alcoholics. Vinegar is also a relatively weak extraction menstruum (solvent) for cannabinoids and essential oils, but it is better at pulling minerals out of herbs. You can also make a blend of any of the three menstruums.

Sublingual sprays became popular in the marketplace because they were modeled on a successful pharmaceutical product made in England called Sativex. They are medicinal oils or alcohol tinctures that you apply by spraying them under the tongue. This encourages absorption through the mucous membranes of the mouth, a rapid onset method of ingestion.

Time of onset: Very rapid for alcohol tinctures. Glycerites and vinegars will be slower as they will go through the digestive system.

Duration of effect: 1–4 hours

Risk of THC overdose: Medium for THC-containing tinctures

Target areas: circulatory system, whole body

Conditions sublingual medicines are ideal for: Most conditions

Katie's Story

The first marijuana medicine I ever made was a tincture. After growing my first patch in 1995, I threw some buds in a jar and covered them with vodka. After a few weeks, I poured some off and tried it. I didn't get high, but I liked the other effects. (Now I realize that there was little THC in the tincture because I hadn't used heat to decarboxylate the THCA.) I strained the rest of the bottle and started handing it out for friends to try.

My friend Jane heard about it and called me one day to ask for some for her partner, Katie. Katie had severe pelvic pain during her periods and often took five or six Vicodin a day during her moonflow. Jane was desperate to help her out, but first she warned me that Katie hadn't smoked pot for years because she no longer liked being high—it had started to make her paranoid.

Katie tried the tincture I provided and got seemingly miraculous results—results she never experienced from smoking the herb. Her initial dose was fifteen drops and it definitely took the edge off of her pain. Then she upped the dose to thirty drops and the pain disappeared altogether.

"It just sort of faded away!" she said, amazed. "And I felt so relaxed that I just fell asleep and slept for four hours."

When her pain crept back in, she took another dose and it worked again. After two months of success, she decided to dose herself between periods as well to see what happened.

"I just took a squirt when I remembered," she admitted, "every couple of days."

This seemed to prevent the premenstrual pain and inflammation and shorten her period. She stuck with this regimen until menopause and never needed another Vicodin.

I, too, was thrilled with the results, but at the same time I thought it odd that smoking pot didn't help with her pain, but a tincture did. I filed it away in my mind for future consideration. Meanwhile I continued to hear about great results from the tincture I'd distributed throughout my community, and I was on my way to becoming a clinical herbalist.

Edibles and Medibles

Food as medicine and medicine as food is the natural way to stay healthy! Eating marijuana is good for you on all levels, from the benefits of eating a green vegetable to balancing the nervous system to healing cancer. And, pot is also an ideal way to treat your upper digestive system and your liver!

Eating uncooked pot—hemp seeds, hemp seed oil, fresh leaves or buds (or fresh-dried leaves or buds)—is a low-risk, highly nutritious way to feed yourself, and you can choose how much THC to include. But that's not what's generally meant by "edibles" or "medibles." Those terms usually refer to food that has been cooked or baked with high-THC pot, and as I've explained elsewhere, when THC goes through the digestive system, the liver breaks it down into metabolites that are up to five times more psychoactive than THC itself. When people overdose on THC, it is usually from eating too many yummy cooked treats with a time of onset that is delayed by hours and has a long duration of effect. Those who overdo an edible will be uncomfortable (but in no danger) for a couple of hours.

However, their long-lasting effect also makes edibles ideal for keeping medicine in your system for extended periods of time so you can sleep, or stay out of pain, or control inflammation or nausea throughout the night.

Time of onset: 1/2 hour–2 hours
Duration of effect: 2–6 hours
Risk of THC overdose: High
Target areas: Digestive system, whole body
Conditions edibles are ideal for: Most conditions that require a long duration of effect like insomnia, digestive system issues, or long hikes in the woods

Capsules and Sprinkles

Capsules and sprinkles can be made from powdered leaves, buds, or roots. They can also include kief (concentrated crystals separated from the plant matter), which is much, much stronger. If there is no decarboxylated THC present, these are not psychoactive. If you don't want them to be psychoactive, do not take THCA sprinkles or capsules with hot food. Sprinkles are a convenient way to include microdoses of marijuana in your meals. Put them on cold dishes if you want them non-psychoactive or in higher amounts in your hot recipes if you want more of a high.

Suppositories

In practice we have discovered many advantages to rectal and vaginal applications of marijuana medicine. Solid or liquid suppositories are ideal for unconscious patients and those with impaired oral ingestion. They are a non-psychoactive way to imbibe THC, so they seem ideal for patients who need very high doses of THC quickly and do not want to take the time to build up a tolerance to its psychoactivity. Unfortunately, there is no useful research being done on rectal or vaginal absorption of cannabis, so we don't know how much reaches the blood system when used this way.

Time of onset: Rapid; 10–15 minutes average

Duration of effect: 4–8 hours; peak at 2–3 hours

Risk of THC overdose: Vaginally, no risk; rectally, extremely low when inserted correctly because the THC never reaches the liver

Target areas: The "nether regions," the colon, rectum, and reproductive regions, low back, hips

Conditions that suppositories are ideal for: Seizures, vomiting, hemorrhoids, vaginal infections, uterine cramps, endometriosis, ovarian cysts, low back pain or disease, hip pain or disease, infertility, cancers and other diseases of the cervix, prostate, rectum, and colon. (Sending medicine through the digestive system, or inhaling it, is clearly a less direct route to these regions.) These applications are ideal for anyone in whom the oral route is impaired, like someone who is fasting before surgery or someone with an esophageal illness. Suppositories are a great treatment for vomiting because they are antiemetic. Cannabis therapy can be administered rectally to an unconscious person or one who has just suffered a stroke or heart attack. Cannabis is neuroprotective and a powerful antioxidant in the brain, so suppositories are an excellent therapy for treating ischemic events. Cannabis medications can be applied this way to stop a seizure, but they are more effective if rubbed on the gums of the patient.

Warning: If a rectal suppository is inserted too high, it can become psychoactive because the hemorrhoidal vein will pick up the THC and carry it directly to the liver, where it will be converted to extremely psychoactive metabolites.

Infused Oils, Butters, and Fats for Internal Use

In addition to topical use, described above, infused oils, butters, or fats can be ingested alone or as the part of any recipe. They can be psychoactive or non-psychoactive depending on the presence of decarboxylated THC. They are good for the digestive system, cancers, anxiety, sleep, pain, and anything else you would consume pot for. For psychoactivity they follow the same guidelines as "medibles."

Concentrates

In addition to the above traditional medicines, we have recently learned how to make ultraconcentrated forms of marijuana medicine. These are extremely potent and can contain anywhere from 50–90 percent cannabinoid content. Their effects are dependent on how they are made and how they are ingested. This revolution in medicine making is thanks to a Canadian named Rick Simpson.

Today there are many kinds of concentrated cannabis medicines available, most of them made with solvents other than alcohol. Not all of them are beneficial, and there are many confusing names and misnomers for concentrates out there. I prefer the term *concentrate* because it is the clearest description and indicates the potency of the medicine. Many cannabis concentrates are made with hydrocarbon solvents like naphtha, butane, or propane. These solvents are petroleum products, and concentrates made using them often contain harmful residuals of the solvent used. This means the client smokes or imbibes the solvent as well as the medicine. They are also dangerous to use at home because the equipment used has the potential to explode!

Many companies are now using carbon dioxide as a solvent, and although these concentrates are cleaner, they require expensive equipment, and the product is often stripped of terpenes. Many concentrates are sold in disposable plastic cartridges to be inhaled through a battery-operated vaporizing pen, and toxic flavoring agents or thinning agents like propylene glycol are often added. The heating element in a vape pen—a metal wire—gets slowly vaporized along with the medicine and enters your lungs. However, vape pens can prove useful when the utmost discretion is needed, such as when traveling, and there are other less toxic vaporizing devices available—do your research before you buy one.

In making concentrates, most home medicine makers prefer to use high proof (150 to 200 proof) food-grade alcohol. Although once limited to grain alcohols like Everclear, now high proof, organic, and biodynamic ethanols are available made from grapes, cane, wheat, and other plants. These solvents are extremely safe to work with when following the simple safety precautions inherent to working with a flammable substance. Using ethanol, we can keep concentrated cannabis medicines in the hands of the people, without reliance on doctors, labs, and pharmacies.

When choosing a concentrated medicine that you have not made yourself, always ask what solvent was used and if the plants were grown outdoors and organically. Cannabis plants are bioaccumulators that draw in any ambient toxins and chemicals in the air and soil (or indoor "bath") and store them in their tissues. If these plants are then concentrated, the medicine will contain the concentrated toxins as well. When you concentrate a plant's medicine, you are also concentrating any pesticide residues, molds, mildews, and even "organic" chemical fertilizer or insect repellents on that plant.

This has been a big problem with CBD medicines derived from "hemp." Industrial hemp has a very low cannabinoid content, and therefore an exponentially larger amount of these plants must be used and an exponentially larger amount of their bioaccumulated toxins is condensed in the medicine. This can cause extreme illness. All herbs grown for medicine should be grown in clean soil, in the sun, with no applications of anything that is harmful to the Earth. Farmers and growers need to commit to making their own soil from natural manures and structural elements, and testing it for heavy metals and other toxins that the plants could pull up through their roots.

Rick Simpson's Story

In 2003 Rick Simpson was diagnosed with basal cell carcinoma skin cancer. He had a lesion surgically removed from his face, but it soon returned, along with two others. Rick remembered hearing on the radio back in the 1970s of a study claiming that THC could kill cancer in mice. He decided to make the strongest possible marijuana medicine. He used 99 percent isopropyl alcohol as a solvent, evaporated it off with heat, and created a tarlike medicine that he applied to one of the spots on his face, bandaged, and left alone for four days. Upon removing the bandage, the cancer had gone and its place was new healthy pink skin.

He then applied it to his other lesions, and they healed too. He tried to share his story with doctors and cancer organizations, but they refused to listen. So, Rick began to hand the medicine out to friends with skin cancer, and they had the same great results.

Soon some folks decided to try taking it orally for their internal cancers. They had to begin with microdoses because the psychoactive level was so high, but if they increased their dosage very slowly they built up a tolerance to that side effect. When they were ingesting about a gram of Simpson Oil a day, they found that their tumors were shrinking, and their cancers were disappearing. Rick continued growing and making his medicine and giving it away. Even after having his home raided multiple times and having over 2,600 cannabis plants cut down and taken by the Canadian government, he continues to produce the oil and help others.

In 2008 filmmaker Christian Laurette released the first documentary on YouTube sharing Rick's story, "Run from the Cure." Since Rick began his journey, he claims to have helped over five thousand people personally with this amazing oil and healed thousands of cancers and other illnesses. Countless others all over the world have heard his story and have been healed. Rick was the inspiration for the Cure Your Own Cancer website—still one of the best resources out there.

Below are some common but *inaccurate* names of cannabis concentrates.

Cannabis oil —This term is too general. A concentrate is not an oil. This term can be confused with a vegetable oil that has been infused with cannabis, which has a much milder potency than a concentrate. Also, this term does not tell us the solvent that was used to manufacture it.

Hemp oil—This term is already in use for the oil that is pressed from the hemp seed, a very different kind of medicine! Again, the solvent is unknown.

CBD oil—CBD concentrate is a far clearer description.

Dab—A concentrate made with hexane, butane, or propane. It is usually "dabbed" onto a smoking device or vaporizer and inhaled. It is often unclean and can retain residual solvent.

Shatter—A concentrate that has had the fats and waxes of the plant removed. Usually made with hexane, propane, or butane. Instead of a sticky or tarlike consistency, it has the consistency of a hard candy that is then "shattered" into small pieces. It is usually smoked or vaporized. It often retains residual solvent.

PSYCHOACTIVITY RANGES FOR THC MEDICINES*

*Because every person has a unique metabolism and each medicine has a unique cannabinoid profile, this chart is only a *guideline*.

PSYCHOACTIVITY	METHOD OF INGESTION	FORM OF THC
The most psychoactive	Consumed concentrates	Extremely high THC metabolites
Extremely psychoactive	Cooked and consumed, such as baked goods, soup, candy	High THC metabolites
Very psychoactive	Hot tea	THC and THC metabolites
Very psychoactive	Smoked or vaporized concentrates	Very high THC
Psychoactive	Smoked or vaporized plant	THC
Psychoactive	Activated tinctures/oils	THC
Psychoactive	Dried and consumed raw powdered, crumbled, soaked in milk, etc.	THC
Not psychoactive (unless a rectal suppository is inserted too high)	Rectal or vaginal suppositories	THC
Not psychoactive	Tinctures of raw and dried, administered orally	No heat has been applied; these are not psychoactive for most
Not psychoactive	Applied topically (any form), such as baths, soaks, salves and infused oils, alcohol tinctures, concentrates	THC
Not psychoactive	Fresh	THC acid only

7

Additional Cannabis
Therapy Tools

BREATHING

Like the endocannabinoid system, breathing is a bridge between body
and spirit, and breathing techniques are used in many spiritualities
as tools for healing. Most Westerners never learn how to breathe correctly, with slow complete inhales and exhales that result in the belly
fully extending and the diaphragm fully contracting and relaxing.
Most spend their lives with shallow, rapid breathing patterns. Shallow
breathing does not fully oxygenate the blood or muscles. It constricts
the stomach, resulting in issues in our digestive tract and enteric nervous system. It keeps our nervous system on high alert. It represses grief,
which gets trapped just below the breast bone. Other factors, such as
slumped posture, or psychological defense mechanisms, prevent normal
breathing as well. Cannabis therapy induces the slow deep breathing
that invites balance and health.

Like cannabis, breathing creates a link between the conscious and
the unconscious and both also balance the central nervous system
(CNS) and the autonomic nervous system (ANS). Inhaling prepares
the body for action, while exhaling relaxes the mind and body. When
our exhale is longer and slower than our inhale, we spend more time
in a relaxed state than in a stimulated state. By consciously controlling

our breathing we can relax our CNS and bring our usually autonomous ANS under our conscious control. We can reverse or prevent the fight-or-flight reaction, control our adrenal glands, heart rate, digestion, and rest cycles. We can bring a runaway stress reaction back under mindful rule.

Cannabis therapy deepens and slows our breathing patterns, which can help us turn off the adrenaline response and infuse more oxygen into the whole body. It can help chronically stressed people experience what *it feels like* to turn off their fight-or-flight response and to understand why that is an important goal.

In addition to anxiety issues, breathing exercises are valuable for pain management, heart strengthening, respiratory issues, grieving, depression, digestion, chronic illnesses, and many other issues.

TRIGGERS AND RESPONSES

Therapy for mental and spiritual disorders often benefits by replacing an unconscious and unhealthy reaction to a trigger with cultivated, healthy responses.

Many patients discover that their triggers revolve around thoughts of the future. Worry and anxiety sit firmly in false predictions of what the future will bring. Because the future occurs only in the imagination, most of the things that people worry about never actually happen. Yet they become stuck in their fears, and being stuck in a stressed state leads to exhaustion, an open door for depression.

For its part, the depressive end of the anxiety spectrum can be rooted in constant ruminations on difficult events in the past. Unfortunately, memories are not good records of our past because they are "colored" by subsequent experiences and so change with each retrieval. To practice coming out of anxiety and/or depression we focus on the present.

"Being present" is one of the most common lessons presented in almost every spiritual philosophy and religion. It is a primary tool for handling stress. When we keep our thoughts and feelings in the present moment, we can let go of our fear of what the future holds and release the emotions associated with old issues. Using spirit-activating marijuana medicines pulls us into the present moment, allowing us to take a break from obsessing over the past or stressing over the future. Carrying something that symbolizes the present with you, like a stone in your pocket, prayer/meditation beads, or a string around your wrist, helps to bring focus to the here and now. Using marijuana, like smoking a CBD joint, is a popular tool for being present.

Recognizing triggers and practicing "being present" (and it is a lifelong practice for most of us mortals) allows us to begin to cultivate desired responses to those triggers to replace the unwanted stress reaction. In essence, we can learn to replace an anxiety attack with healthier behavior. When developing chosen responses to a trigger, the usual first step is slow deep breathing to prevent the sympathetic nervous system from taking over. Breath is a tool we always have with us, and if we can control our breathing, we can bring our nervous system under control. Then we can introduce and practice a chosen behavioral response.

"How do you want to respond when a car backfires in the street?" "How do you want to feel when you see your ex in the grocery store?" "What do you want to do when that memory comes up?" These are typical questions to help clients create their new behavior. When they have crafted their responses, they practice them in therapy until they become automatic, like practicing scales on a piano.

FLOWER ESSENCES

Flower essences, or flower remedies, are powerful tools for working with emotional imbalance. Often called energetic or vibrational medicine, flower essences resonate with the energetic vibrational patterns of animals, like two wavelengths entraining. We use flower remedies to catalyze changes in our deep emotional state and to shift the spiritual state subtly and profoundly.

They are made by infusing the energy of flowers (or other parts of a plant) in water, which is then potentized through a series of dilutions, similar to a homeopathic remedy, and then the energy is stabilized by adding alcohol. Every plant has its own unique vibrational energetic pattern and healing qualities. We can use these potions to "wake up" deeply buried emotions, inspire an infusion of positive emotions, and clear out old, stuck emotions. When formulated together, they provide a complex, deep, and subtle shift in healing.

I often formulate flower essences that people (or animals) can use to calm the symptoms of anxiety. When I make some essences, I take them a step further so that they also resonate at the spiritual level. For example, my ganja essences help people connect with their true selves, so we can begin to discover the root causes of their condition. To quote Dr. Christiane Northrup, "The most wonderful thing about flower essences is their ability to promote healing on the emotional, mental, and spiritual levels."*

AROMATHERAPY

There is no denying that aromas have the power to shift our emotional state. The smell of cookies baking can make you miss Grandma, a bouquet of flowers can shift a girlfriend's anger, a lavender-perfumed handkerchief can soothe a widow at her husband's funeral. Fragrances can be calming, uplifting, stimulating, grounding, or sedating, and they can provide clarity or have a combination of effects. Some aromas can even invoke dreams.

Aromatherapy is the holistic science of essential oils, the tiny volatile molecules responsible for plant aromas. Essential oils are a very strong concentration of aromatic plant chemicals that include terpenes and phenols. These oils pass right through the blood-brain barrier and directly

---

*Christiane Northrup, M.D., is a visionary pioneer and a leading authority in the field of women's health and wellness, which includes the unity of mind, body, emotions, and spirit. She is a board-certified OB/GYN physician, a multiple *New York Times* bestselling author, and has hosted many television specials. Her eight books include *Women's Bodies, Women's Wisdom, The Wisdom of Menopause,* and her most recent, *Dodging Energy Vampires.*

modulate the biological factors involved with stress, including heart rate, blood pressure, and immune function. They encourage deep breathing, balance the nervous system, and bring us into the present moment.

The same aroma can affect people differently. A restless person may feel calm after inhaling the aroma of lavender, while someone who is feeling low may get an uplifting and invigorating feeling from the same scent. We refer to some essential oils as "adaptogens" because they can literally "adapt" to the needs of the person using the oil.

Aromatherapy is a profound tool for anxiety. These medicines can quickly quell an anxious reaction. Used regularly, they can keep our mental and emotional states in balance, while protecting us from infectious disease. Some aromas that can relieve anxiety include lavender, lemon balm, chamomile, geranium, frankincense, vetiver, pine, fir, cedar, grapefruit, orange, and lemon.

The simplest way to use aromatherapy is to stop and smell the plants around you.

At one point, when merely opening my appointment book became a trigger for stress, I started keeping a rose geranium leaf in the book. Now I look forward to opening the book, smelling that aroma, and remembering to do some deep breathing. The aromatic herbs that line the pathways of my healing center release their aromas when clients brush by, encouraging people to slow down and breathe. One of the great lessons that anxiety disorders teach us is to slow down, be present, and smell the roses. Using marijuana and walking in an aromatic forest combines exercise, deep breathing, a connection with nature, and aromatherapy for a complete holistic therapy.

Since life is not always full of flowers, we can create small medicines to carry with us. A small sachet of posies in our pocket, or some essential oil on a handkerchief or scarf, can carry us through a stressful event. I also make aromatherapy spritzer bottles and roller balls small enough to keep handy in a pocket, purse, or car. These are all excellent and immediate responses to a stress trigger. Alternatively, aromatherapy can augment yoga, meditation, baths, foot soaks, or any other anxiety therapy one might use.

It takes a tremendous amount of an herb to distill a tiny amount of essential oil. For example, it takes about three pounds of lavender flowers to produce around 15 ml of lavender essential oil, 242,000 rose petals produce approximately 5 ml of rose essential oil, and approximately 6,000 pounds of lemon balm produce just a single pound of essential oil. As you can imagine, cannabis essential oil has not yet found a market.

It is easy, however, to make small batches of hydrosol from pot's fresh leaves, flowers, and roots. You can make your own steam or water distillation on your stovetop or with an electric water distiller. Hydrosols contain many essential oils and some of the water-soluble constituents of an herb.

Most of the terpenes and phenols found in cannabis essential oils are also in other, more accessible plants. For example, we find caryophyllene in hops, clove, and rosemary essential oil and pinene in conifer and sage essential oils. You can purchase these inexpensive essential oils from health food stores and herb shops, but be sure to find organic products as any pesticides present in the plant will be concentrated in the oil too.

Warning: Many essential oils are so strong that they will burn the skin. You cannot dilute or wash away essential oils with water. Always dilute essential oils into a carrier oil, even when dropping them into a whole tub of water for a bath or foot soak. Always shake spritzers that contain essential oils immediately before spraying them.

DIET, EXERCISE, AND REST

Let food be thy medicine and medicine be thy food.

HIPPOCRATES

A proper diet and getting enough exercise and rest are major components of health care, and marijuana medicine enhances all three. These tools are particularly important for anyone suffering from illness and/or anxiety because they help bring the autonomous nervous system under more conscious control.

Our ancestors regularly consumed the herbs and mushrooms they gathered for food. All of these had medicinal benefits. This is the way our bodies are best adapted to taking in medicine. It is far better to heal ourselves with teas and food than with supplements or pharmaceutical drugs. A diverse diet is key to ensure that we consume a full range of tonic medicine and nutrients. Weed, like all herbs, works better in recipes with other herbs and foods.

A caffeine-free diet is almost essential when battling insomnia or any issue that has anxiety as a symptom because caffeine initiates the very flight-or-fight reaction that we are trying to stop. Switching from coffee and caffeinated teas to herbal teas made with CBD-rich pot leaves is a huge step toward taking conscious control of your nervous system. So is a diet that is high in protein and oils and low in carbohydrates. People on constant alert burn through carbs very rapidly and can suffer swings in blood sugar and mood because of it. Eating small amounts of protein throughout the day prevents low blood sugar episodes that can trigger anxiety or cause one to become "hangry" or angry due to hunger. Hemp seeds are tasty, high-protein treats that you can sprinkle on most any food or mix into any recipe.

We need enough balanced essential fatty acids and cholesterol in the diet to avoid dry tissues and to form the strong myelin sheaths that insulate and protect the nerves. Hemp seed oil (often called hemp oil) is the best source for perfectly balanced omega-3 and omega-6 fatty acids. I make many recipes that combine hemp seeds, hemp seed oil, hemp leaves, and other adaptogenic and nervine herbs. They are tasty treats that heal cancer, skin issues, nervous system problems, and prevent anxiety issues!

When stress or anxiety trigger a fight-or-flight reaction, it should be followed by exercise. After all, that is what the reaction is designed for. If we don't use up the adrenalin (epinephrine) and blood sugar released during an episode, it will begin to cause oxidative damage. Regular exercise encourages deep breathing, relieves stress, relaxes the muscles, keeps the nervous system in balance, boosts immunity, and strengthens the cardiovascular system. Many people use ganja to enhance their exercise routines. She can increase focus, prevent boredom, decrease pain and inflammation, and help us recover faster from a workout.

Exercise also prepares us for rest and improves sleep. So does ganja. Deep rest and sleep (two different things) are a necessary part of therapy for all illnesses. Without them, our systems cannot recover from the overstimulation and oxidative damage caused by the illness, and we will become drained and exhausted.

In addition, everyone needs daily periods of nonsleeping rest. A time that they can "space out" mentally and emotionally for recovery and to build resiliency. Some people need strict ritual and routine in their lives so that they can free up their mental space from making and analyzing the frequent decisions and problem-solving needed to get through a day. Others need daily periods of captivating mental stimulation like studying, video games, movies, or puzzles to clear their minds of everyday worries. Others respond best to physical therapies such as exercise, movement meditations, yoga, hot herbal baths, or self-massage with herbal oils. Everyone benefits from time in nature. Creative outlets like art, music, cooking, gardening, or other hobbies that fully engross the attention for blocks of time are popular ways to process stress. Naps during the day are natural and beneficial. Pot can enhance all these activities. Regular ganja breaks, be they psychoactive or just relaxing, provide routine restorative periods that keep us mentally, physically, and spiritually healthy. (In the United States it is traditional among pot smokers to take their break at 4:20 in the afternoon.)

It is difficult for someone who has been in an extended state of excitement to slow down. Weed helps people relax and be still. Pot is a nervine and an adaptogen. Nervines are plant remedies that have a beneficial effect on the nervous system and can act as tonics, stimulants, or relaxants. Adaptogens help us adapt to stress. Often chronic anxiety comes paired with insomnia because the autonomic nervous system has difficulties shifting from the sympathetic (stimulating) to the parasympathetic (rest and digest) nervous system. Dope can help prepare the mind and body for deep sleep. Blended with other calming nervines in a tincture, cannabis can be kept by the bedside and used for interrupted sleep as well.

In sum, inviting non-psychoactive cannabis, like fresh greens, hemp seeds, or CBD tea, into our regular diet helps maintain balance in our nervous systems. Mind-altering cannabis can augment spiritual experiences, exercise, or yoga. A little edible at night can help your rest and increase our recovery rate.

Creating a holistic, flexible cannabis therapy plan involves multiple factors. A full medical, emotional, and spiritual intake is the first step. Then, take into account phytocannabinoid ratios, the biphasic effect of marijuana, the effects of different kinds of medicines, and initial and dynamic dosing to create a menu of possibilities for your patients or clients so that they can choose what is right for their lifestyle and condition. Then, if at all possible, make your own marijuana medicines!

8

Developing a Cannabis Therapy Plan

I wrote this chapter for all readers and clinical healers who want to design holistic cannabis therapy plans for themselves or their clients. This includes physicians, acupuncturists, nurses, massage therapists, mental health practitioners, clinical herbalists, religious leaders, addiction counselors, spiritual healers, veterinarians, animal healers, and others.

Guiding yourself or someone else toward a treatment plan involves looking at a multitude of complex, interrelated factors because not only are we whole beings, but cannabis is a holistic medicine. The beauty of this intelligent plant is that she "first does no harm" so that we can safely experiment to find the plan that is right for ourselves or others without fear.

The complexity of cannabis therapy often confuses the general public, and so they are seeking out educated and experienced cannabis therapy consultants to help them figure out what kind of medicine is best for them. As a consultant, you may or may not be a clinical healer, but you should be able to provide advice about marijuana's psychoactivity levels, various methods of ingestion and application, and antidotes for THC overdoses, as well as the importance of whole plant medicine. It helps to know how to blend cannabis with other medicinal herbs in food and formulas, how to make marijuana medicines, which parts of the plant contain which chemicals, and what parts of the body, mind, or spirit to target in common conditions and ailments.

Consultants should start by exploring and researching a client's list of physical, mental, emotional, and spiritual issues as well as the connections between them. I have never in my practice encountered a person with only one ailment. For example, they may come asking about insomnia, but soon we find that there is also a kidney issue, a "bad back," an unhappy marriage, and/or a schedule that leaves no time for rest. While it is true that offering someone a salve for their arthritic knee can work a small miracle for their pain and mobility, and a CBD tincture might prevent someone's migraines, when we match one medicine with one symptom, we are using only a tiny bit of this mighty plant's power to help only a small part of a whole person.

Herbology teaches that a specific dosage of one herb is not right for everyone with a similar issue. Your colitis is different from her colitis because you are different from her. You may run hot while she runs cold. You might have tremendous stress in your life right now, while she has thyroid issues. You are seventy-two and smoked cigarettes for fifty years. She is seventeen and in love for the first time. Should you both use the same dosages of the same medicine? PTSD involves the mind, body, and spirit, so how could the treatment not? How can a treatment plan, designed for one unique soul, suit another? All individuals seeking healing have unique stress reactions, physical challenges, lifestyles, and abilities that determine their therapy choices. Exploring these circumstances is an essential step in putting together a cannabis treatment plan.

Once we understand our clients as whole beings, then we begin our research. We must account for the myriad of functions found in the endocannabinoid system and consider phytocannabinoids, essential oils, terpenes, flavonoids, alkaloids and other beneficial plant compounds, their locations in the plant, and their synergistic effects when they work together. We can then provide a menu of cannabis medicines that might help them out and let them choose from the menu what is right for their lifestyle and condition. It is also extremely helpful to be able to tell them how to make any medicines that are not available or that are too expensive to purchase.

My aim in this chapter is to shine a light on important considerations when formulating a treatment plan for yourself, your animals, or others. I discuss the importance of listening as a first step, and I explore the effects of different phytocannabinoid ratios, the biphasic effect of medicine, how different kinds of medicines invoke different reactions, and help clear up some of the complex, confusing decisions involved in dosing. We will consider as well information already touched upon in this book, such as issues involved in introducing new users to THC and what to do in cases of "overmedication."

Amelia's Story

Amelia is a fifty-six-year-old bookkeeper who originally came to me for help with kidney issues. When she developed kidney stones in 1992, she had them "blasted," as she called it, with lithotripsy. After a long recovery, she discovered that one kidney had developed scar tissue and was reduced to 50 percent of its function. She also had a parathyroid tumor that had been stable for the past ten years. She was interested in natural therapies that might boost her kidney function and support her endocrine system.

A nonholistic healer might have simply recommended herbal teas and medicine for the kidneys and endocrine system and not delved further. However, as we continued to talk, Amelia admitted that she probably "ruined" her kidneys when she was bulimic for twenty years. And that she was having frequent, severe anxiety attacks. And that she was deeply grieving her dog who had died recently. And that when she was young, she had been drugged, kidnapped, and raped for a week before escaping. She was also chronically constipated, anemic, and felt that she drank too much wine.

There was more, of course, and as we worked together over the months it became clear to me how all the symptoms were interrelated and where the core problems lay.

We started by tackling her immediate anxiety symptoms and reactions. With basic breathing exercises and a cannabis-based antianxiety formula, she reported back after two weeks that she was having far fewer incidents devolve into full-blown anxiety attacks and that her consumption of wine had been reduced by half, because she reached for the tincture and did some deep breathing before opening the wine. She had never regained an appetite even though her bulimia had subsided when she met her current partner years ago, but now she reported having a slightly better appetite and even gaining a little weight.

I continued adding different types of therapy every couple of weeks and she continued to improve greatly. We added aromatherapy with terpenes from cannabis and other herbs for use when she felt triggered. She placed an altar on her kitchen table, and we designed a premeal ritual to begin consciously honoring food again. She began using an herbal bitters formula with cannabis to stimulate her digestive juices and boost her appetite. She would take a few minutes to sit at the altar and do some deep breathing before eating to try to consciously move into the "rest and digest" part of her nervous system. She loved the CBD chai herbal tea I blended for her, and she drank it after eating to calm her and to warm up her gut and bring in circulation for better digestion. She moved from eating at her desk all the time to setting the table and enjoying a meal with her partner.

TAKING THE FIRST STEP: LISTENING

The first, and often the most important, healing act that we can offer someone is to listen. Many who come to me have never been truly heard before. Or harsher than that, they have been invalidated, told that they were crazy, or lying, or worse. Their feelings of desperation and isolation have been discounted, and often they are shamed for claiming that marijuana helps them.

Merely by allowing them to speak their story, their full story, they can begin to break down the dam holding in their dis-ease, and healing energy can begin to flow (often in the form of tears). They may have seen dozens of doctors and pharmacists over a period of decades but have never been asked, "But how do you feel about this? What do you think? What have you tried before? What helped? What didn't? What other issues do you face that might be related? Is the onset of this condition related to a traumatic event or a change in your lifestyle? What are your healing goals? What is your perspective in life?"

When given a chance to explore and share themselves, people can become their own best doctors. In the end they can often clearly tell me what they need to heal, and I am left as merely a guide to present options and help them choose a path to health. I have never been in a position of knowing what a person needs better than they do themselves. Thank the Goddess for that!

ADDRESSING THE FEAR FACTOR

For Americans especially, there are a lot of ways that fear creeps into using cannabis. Many in Western society have been taught to fear the "devil weed." Although the Western world has been brainwashed by the U.S. government to fear this plant and forced to give it up, in fact society has been misled and lied to. However, the campaigns against pot have engendered social fear, fear of prosecution, fear of being drug tested, and fear of judgment. There is fear that pot is damaging and causes psychosis or paranoia. There is fear of helicopters and violent police actions against users or that their children will be taken away from them. There is fear that this illegal plant is the only hope to survive cancer, and fear that if this plant is taken away, parents will watch their child have seizures two hundred times a day. These are all real fears! If you or anyone you are working with experiences any of these fears, they need to be addressed as part of the cannabis therapy plan, so they don't interfere with the therapy.

To work with someone who is afraid of pot, begin by asking them about their previous experiences with the herb and listen to their story. Find out what their fear stems from and address the cause. Is the fear of THC or of the whole plant? If it's the plant, start by introducing topical medicines or put some leaves in a foot soak. If they pray or meditate, have them begin to include the plant in their ruminations. I've found that hemp seeds or sprouts, raw cannabis infused in honey, and sun tea are all good ways to introduce someone to ingesting hemp. For fear of THC, see "Dosing" later in this chapter for guidance in introducing psychoactive medications.

In all cases, only individuals know if cannabis is the best medicine for them or not. We are all our own best doctors and even if you think you "know" what someone needs, trust me—you don't! You can only help them discover that for themselves. Fear of cannabis is usually rooted in ignorance. Help empower yourself and others with the truth. Create awareness. Knowing the truth shall set us and this plant free!

CONSIDER ANXIETY LEVELS

THC medicine can hinder or help someone with anxiety—depending on the dose, the formula, and the individual's response. Because THC can raise the heart rate, it is a bit of a wild card for individuals with problem anxiety reactions, so it is best to start with a very low-THC or THC-free medicine.

There are many options (see "Types of Marijuana Medicine," chapter 6), such as fresh marijuana, a strain or medicine with a high ratio of CBD to THC, or a nondecarboxylated medicine high in THCA and very low in THC. CBD is anxiolytic (relaxing), and modulates the stimulating properties of THC, so I usually recommend including it when dealing with anxiety. Some terpenes in pot are stimulating, like limonene, so start out by avoiding those and using weed with sedating terpenes like myrcene or balancing terpenes like linalool.

Since clients with anxiety disorders are some of the most sensitive cases relating to THC medicines, they do best with accompanying counseling and close monitoring as we investigate their responses to THC. That said, for many people inhaling THC is an immediate aid in slowing or stopping the anxiety reaction, and it can even become a cultivated response in the tool box when triggers arise.

Cannabis therapy can not only relieve anxiety symptoms it can also help one discover their causes and in some cases help to heal the condition. However, that calls for a well-designed therapy plan with a multipronged approach including counseling.

> *Hashish will be, indeed, for the impressions and familiar thoughts of the man, a mirror which magnifies, yet no more than a mirror.*
>
> CHARLES BAUDELAIRE, "THE POEM OF HASHISH"
> IN *ARTIFICIAL PARADISE*

THC AND CBD RATIOS

As people become more knowledgeable about cannabis, their next question is usually about the differences between THC and CBD, and what ratio might be best for them. Phytocannabinoid ratios of a plant are initially determined by a lab. If a clone is made from a "mother plant" it will retain the identical cannabinoid ratio. A plant raised from seed usually needs to be tested.

A ratio gives no indication of the strength, or potency, of a cannabinoid in a plant, it just tells you how much of a cannabinoid is present compared to all the other cannabinoids measured. A 4:1 THC:CBD ratio means that for every four parts of THC in that plant, there is one part of CBD. For example, for every 4 milligrams (mgs) of THC there is 1 mg of CBD. To repeat, a ratio does not tell you how strong a medicine is, i.e., how many mg of THC a medicine or plant contains. A ratio does not tell you how many milligrams of THC there are in your 4:1 brownie!

Each individual reacts to cannabis differently, but because these cannabinoids do have original and unique benefits from each other, different ratios have different effects. It is usually best to include both together in a treatment plan because they both strengthen each other and balance each other out. Sometimes a THC-dominant dosage is preferable and sometimes a CBD-dominant dosage is better. For example, in the case of childhood seizure disorders, people found a very high CBD/low THC ratio extremely effective in reducing the number and severity of seizures. According to Project CBD, severe childhood epileptics who are given CBD oil products experience a near complete cessation of seizures; most experience a decrease of seizures. However, for some children, CBD worsens the condition. When parents add a low level of THC or THCA to the medicine, they may see the changes they are seeking.

For another example, a high-THC medicine can aggravate psychosis, but a high CBD ratio is considered antipsychotic. As we will discuss later, when determining initial dosages for nontopical cannabis it is always best to go "low and slow." Start with a low dose, evaluate the effect, then increase the dose slowly until the desired effect is achieved.

So, be careful when considering recommendations that determine specific ratios of phytocannabinoids for specific diseases or symptoms. They are based on the "treat the disease and not the individual" approach. Project CBD explains it best:

> [Cannabis] is personalized medicine. . . . A person's sensitivity to THC is a key factor in determining the appropriate ratio and dosage of CBD-rich medicine. . . . CBD can lessen or neutralize the intoxicating effects of THC. So, a greater ratio of CBD-to-THC means less of a high. . . . Those who don't like THC have the option of healing without the high by using a CBD-rich remedy with only a small amount of THC. But a low THC remedy, while not intoxicating, is not always the most effective treatment option. In essence, the goal is to administer measurable doses of a CBD-rich remedy that includes as much THC as a person is comfortable with."[1]

Assess the effects, and modify dosages accordingly. Remember that people build up tolerances to THC, so more can be added every 3–4 days.

BIPHASIC EFFECTS

Another little-known and confusing action of ganja is that she often has a different effect on the same person at different dosages. For example, a small dose of THC can be stimulating, while a large dose can help someone to sleep. This is an example of a biphasic effect, which means that an herb can have opposite effects depending on the person using it, the dosage, the ratio of cannabinoids, the setting, tolerance, and other factors. For example, lots of people smoke THC-rich pot to help them relax and drift into sleep. The same pot will perk up others. A small dose of THC can trigger some people's sympathetic nervous systems and make them feel anxious, but a large dose can activate their parasympathetic nervous systems and promote deep, dreamless sleep. In private marijuana may relax you, but in public it may make you feel nervous. Often, a consistent dose of a consistent strain will bring about desired effects for a given time and then stop working due to a buildup of tolerance, and you might need to try another strain or ratio to recapture the effect you are looking for. The biphasic effects of cannabis are part of why therapy plans need to be personal and dynamic.

FORMING A DYNAMIC PLAN

So how do we form a holistic cannabis therapy plan for ourselves or another individual? A good plan will be flexible so it can change as needed, will target the whole person or animal, and will consist of more than one type of cannabis medicine and include complementary herbs. We need a dynamic process to determine dosage, taking into consideration initial doses and how to increase or decrease them. We will consider all methods of ingestion, psychoactivity levels, and how to target areas of the body, emotional states, mental states, and spiritual practices. We basically want to present a salad bar of different medicines to someone so they can build their own ideal salad at each meal.

It is important to realize that while seeking whole plant medicine, the whole plant doesn't have to be present in every medicine. If someone is using a CBD oil without THC for seizures, he or she can use a tincture with THC or vaporize a THC strain to complement it. If someone is taking a high-THC Simpson Oil for cancer, that person may want to also consume a CBD edible to add its anticancer powers to the mix . . . or to balance out the psychoactive or anxiogenic effects of THC, or to help alleviate the stress of being sick, or so on!

If individuals are taking a CBD medicine for its anti-inflammatory effect, they might also want to include a THCA-rich juice or salad dressing in their daily diets as well, to take advantage of the combined anti-inflammatory effects of CBD and THCA. People who suffer from anxiety might see better results with a higher dose of CBD than THC in their plan. They may want to smoke a strain with a calming terpene profile and/or include some CBN for its sedative value.

Those with chronic pain and fears about "getting high" might want to start out with some fresh cannabis leaves in a smoothie or sun tea. People who dislike being stoned may want to use their THC strain at night, when they can sleep through the high. Others prefer the lift THC gives them in the morning and use a CBD strain at night to sleep.

DOSING

Because weed is such a personalized medicine, effective dosages are as individual as people are, and they can change throughout the healing process. Let's look at some important factors involved with dosing marijuana medicine.

First, I want to address the word *overdose*. When people hear this phrase, their first impression is that of death, and that has never happened with marijuana. Unlike opioid receptors, there are no cannabinoid receptors within the area of the brain that regulates your breathing, so taking too much will never kill you. A much more accurate term is *overmedicated*, and it only applies to high-THC medicines because THC is the only molecule out of hundreds in the plant that can cause that unpleasant reaction when too much is taken. Overmedicating on THC triggers a very uncomfortable response, but it rarely leads to anything more than deep sleep. The most severe cases will involve loss of balance, inability to stand or walk, the spins, vomiting, and a potential for dehydration. Perhaps the equivalent of the aftermath of a night at a college frat party.

If someone has overmedicated on THC, using CBD can reduce the unwanted effects measurably. Whenever clients are consuming a high-THC medicine, I encourage them to keep a fast-acting, high-CBD medicine, like a joint or an alcohol tincture, close by as an antidote. More ancient antidotes include caffeine, lemon juice, and black pepper. Eat too many majoons in Morocco? They will give you a glass of lemonade with a sprinkle of pepper. Drink too much bhang in India? You will be offered a cup of black tea with lemon.

However safe and temporary they are, the effects of overmedicating are miserable and best avoided, especially in someone who is already extremely ill. The important factors to understand are that different forms of high-THC marijuana medicine have different potentials for overmedication, and that it is possible to build up a tolerance to this particular effect of THC while still responding to its other medicinal effects.

The danger factor here has to do with how and when THC is processed by your liver. THC only goes through the liver when it is taken orally and then goes through the digestive system—i.e., when you eat or drink it. This means that the risk of overdose for all other methods of THC application is very low to zero.

THC is converted in the liver to a metabolite called 11-hydroxy-THC, a molecule that is five times more powerful than THC. That means that a 10 mg dose of THC will grow to a 50 mg dose within about ninety minutes of consumption. This difference in physiological response is the biggest risk factor for exceeding your limits. Even habitual smokers and inhalers are often taken by surprise by the effects from consuming THC. These effects are further compounded when mixed with alcohol, and for that reason many people have developed a lifelong fear of marijuana, because they ate "that pot brownie" at a keg party in college.

What to Do if You Do Overdo

Remember, there is no true danger.

Use your CBD antidote.

Drink water.

Call a friend who would understand.

Make a cup of black tea with lemon and a shake of black pepper.

Plug in a funny movie.

Drink more water.

Take Rescue Remedy.

Step outside.

Soak in hot water.

Try to sleep.

Given individual uniqueness, there is no such thing as a "right dose." And there is certainly no such thing as the right dose for a given condition. A small dose of CBD may reduce the pain in your knee, but a large dose might not work at all. One person may stem their bipolar cycles by microdosing with one inhalation of a balanced CBD/THC strain of cannabis, but if they consume an edible, it may aggravate their cycle for days. Once again, each person must be treated as an individual, and therapists can only act as guides as clients determine the correct dosages for themselves.

Because weed is so safe, everyone can experiment to find their right dose by starting with an initial dose of any form of cannabis medicine, evaluating the effects, and adjusting from there.

When using any herbal remedy for the first time, we always "start low and go slow." This means the initial dose should be very low, and dosage increases should be small and happen over a period of days until the desired effects are achieved. In many cases, people or animals only need a microdose of an herb to effectively rebalance their health. Perhaps chewing on a few green leaves or hemp seed sprouts, or taking one drop of a tincture or one small hit off a joint is all that is needed each day to feel better. Start small; wait long enough to ensure that all of the effects have peaked; evaluate the effects. If there's no relief, or not enough, then increase the dose a little bit or add a small dose of a different kind of ganja medicine and reevaluate. Some people need 1,000 mg of CBD to alleviate their pain or anxiety, but others may need only 5 mg. Cannabinoids can make effective changes in a person's system at nanomolar concentrations (an extremely tiny amount), because that is the level at which that person's endocannabinoid system operates.

In the cannabis industry, dosage recommendations revolve around the consumption of THC and, more recently, CBD and other cannabinoids. Dosage recommendations in the industry relate to only one tiny aspect of whole plant medicine—getting high—but they are helpful in working out an initial dosage without overmedicating.

If I need to generalize here, I can say that an initial dose of THC that is safe for most adults to consume without becoming too stoned is 5 mgs. (Of course, a medicine that includes CBD will reduce the risk of getting too high because CBD—and other plant chemicals—modulates the psychoactive effect of THC.) If possible, establish an initial dose of THC by smoking, vaporizing, or using an alcohol tincture. The results of these methods are immediate, clear quickly, and the risk of overdose is almost zero. Whereas the results from eating THC can take up to two hours to peak, last a long time, and are much stronger. If a new user wants to begin with an edible, however, aim for a 5 mg dose of THC or lower. The state of Colorado arbitrarily assigned 10 mg of THC as a "dose" but did not differentiate between smoking or eating that dose. For many elders and new users, smoking those 10 mg would not be a problem, but eating it will knock them for a loop.

The good news is that if one needs to consume large amounts of THC for medical reasons, it is possible to slowly build up a tolerance. Often cancer patients want to take large amounts of high-THC cannabis concentrates to heal their cancer. When starting their regimen, they may only be able to tolerate 10 mg of THC daily. But by continuing with this initial dose, they will be able to double it to 10 mg twice a day within three to four days, because they are getting used to it. After another four days, they can up the dose another 10 mg. By continuing with these low and slow increases, they might be able to consume 500 mg, or even 1,000 mg, per day within a month.

A note on tolerance: Sometimes habitual users develop a tolerance to one of the non-psychoactive medicinal effects of their THC pot. Their pot may no longer be helping them with depression, for instance. In this case, they can regain a therapeutic effect by taking a break for a few days, or by changing strains, ratios, type of medicine, or their method of ingestion. Keeping a therapy plan dynamic improves and extends its effectiveness.

People and animals are evolving, complex, and whole beings made up of a body, a mind, and a spirit. Pot plants are the same. Combining them in a therapy plan must reflect this. To form a plan is really to create a list of options and choose the ones that work best for each individual. The list should include different medicines, parts of the plant, ingestion methods, dosages, and cannabinoid ratios. Once the first few doses have been taken, we evaluate the effects and adapt the plan accordingly. Cannabis therapy, as with all natural therapies, is ever-changing and easily adapts as the individual adjusts throughout the healing journey.

Diana's Story

Diana, a fifty-four-year-old winery employee, suffered chronic pain in her right knee due to an old skiing injury. She worked on a concrete floor and by the end of her shift, the knee would be swollen and the pain nearly unbearable. She had worked her way up from ibuprofen to prescription opiates and soon became addicted. She was worried that she would soon be unable to work. At the first mention of cannabis therapy, her reaction was, "No way! I don't want to be a pothead!" So, we started with some simple changes in her nighttime routine. When she got home, she would ice her knee for twenty minutes. Then she would take a bath using the bath bags I prepared for her containing Epsom salts, cannabis leaves, chamomile flowers, and lavender flowers. After her bath she would ice her knee one more time before bed. After three days she noticed that the inflammation at night was reduced and the pain was starting later during her work shift. She was also sleeping a lot better. Then I gave her a topical salve with cannabis, calendula, comfrey, and St. John's wort to apply when needed. If she used it at work when the pain started, it would back off a few more hours. Then I recommended applying it before the pain started, and that worked even better. From there we began to work with the opiate addiction. Most people who start using cannabis are able to greatly reduce their opiate use, and Diane was no exception. She began using a non-psychoactive cannabis tincture, and as she increased her dosage, she was able to simultaneously decrease her opiate intake until she got off them altogether. I also encouraged her to shorten her work shifts on concrete from 8 hours to 6.5 hours. When she maintains this regimen, she can manage her knee pain. When she "relaxes" her routine, her knee lets her know about it, and that encourages her to stick to it!

9

How to Make Medicine with Marijuana

There are a thousand good reasons to make your own medicine, but here are some of my motivations.

You Are in Charge: Marijuana is first and foremost a medicine by, for, and of the people. When she has been withheld from the people by the powers in control, it hasn't gone well. In the United States and the Western world, prohibition of pot has led to dependence on harmful and often prohibitively expensive pharmaceutical drugs that require the production of, use, and elimination of thousands of harmful chemicals that go on to pollute our water, land, and air. Even now, the newly legal cannabis industry is being taken over by corporations more interested in profit than in health. Making one's own medicine does an end run around corporate medicine.

You Save Money: As of this writing, people are paying about $150 for a vial of CBD oil at a dispensary that they can make for $50 at home. If you can grow your own plant somewhere, the pot-based medicines you make will be even cheaper. Like one of my favorite herbal teachers used to say, "Pick your own damn dandelions!"

It Is Easy: You can make your own medicines with equipment and materials that most folks already have in their kitchen, and the instructions are no more difficult to follow than recipes in cookbooks.

Better Quality: Homemade medicines are of higher quality. When you make your own medicine, you control the ingredients and can use organic, sun-grown herbs and the best organic oils and alcohols. You can avoid petroleum-based waxes and salves and use beeswax instead. You can ensure the quality of the water in your tinctures by using clean, nonchlorinated spring water or well water.

More Power: Homemade medicines can become more powerful with a little magic. You can clean and clear your medicine-making space of bacteria, microbes, funguses, and bad energy with herbal incense and smudge sticks. You can set your intention to make powerful medicine, put your love and healing energy into the medicine, and even tell the medicine what you want it to do. You can bless it or ask your favorite goddess, angel, or spiritual being to bless it. You can incorporate healing crystals and other magical objects into the medicine. You can craft it according to the phases of the moon or the astrological cycles. You can pray or meditate over it. You have this power and Mary Jane loves it! She prefers to work as a team.

Better Flavor: Homemade medicine tastes better! I learned a long time ago that it is one thing to go to the trouble to grow and make medicine and quite another to get people to take it. Make it taste good and you will look forward to your daily doses. Blend your pot into a favorite tea blend, add fruit and sweet herbs like licorice root or stevia to tinctures, or infuse your weed into honey to add to any beverage. Smokable, aromatic herbs like lavender or mugwort can be added to a joint, and tasty herbs like peppermint, cinnamon, or orange peel can go into infused oils. Marijuana syrups and tinctures can make a stellar addition to a cocktail. You can infuse your weed into wine or beer. The possibilities are as endless as your culinary creativity.

It Is Fun: Making your own medicine is simply beautiful. I often joke with my students that the whole reason I got into chemistry and medicine making was the pretty little bottles filled with colorful medicines. You can express your creativity by making your own labels.

A Great Activity for Kids: Just as we need to teach children how to prepare healthy foods and keep a clean kitchen, we can teach them to prepare the household medicine chest. Children love to help make potions and lotions and magic formulas. And they can be learning math, science, and health while playing in the kitchen.

Value-added Products for Farmers: If you are working in the latest trend of farm-to-table food or community supported agriculture, you can add a simple value-added product to your farm. A tea blend, an infused honey, or a vinegar tincture can go a long way to bring in more profit and educate your consumers.

Tradition: Although my husband claims that tradition is just "peer pressure from dead people," in this case I encourage listening to your ancestors! By preparing herbal remedies for yourself and your clients, friends, and family, you are continuing a long tradition because all cultures have traditionally used herbs for food and medicine. If it didn't work, you wouldn't be here!

So, gather your materials, cleanse your kitchen, and commence playing with plants! You are empowering yourself and encouraging your community to gain more self-sufficiency.

DIY: FOOD AS MEDICINE

In chapter 3, "Whole Plant Medicines," I outlined the uses of teas, liniments, salves, and so on. In chapter 6, I discussed the attributes of each type of medicine. Here I go into detail about how to make all those medicines.

How Women Practice Science

Her observations are of nature.
Her research is done gossiping at the well.
Her experiments are stirred up over the stove,
with a baby on her hip.
Her reports are stories over tea.

Her evidence is ten generations of family lore, and from her
well-honed intuition when a hypothesis rises, she takes it right
to the source. She asks the plant, the Earth, her ancestors, her
goddess, her inner self. And, she listens for her teachers' reply.

Her proof comes as a knowing, on the inside. Her theories
are developed based on faith, and all of her potions pass first
through her own lips before trickling down to others.

Her prayers and intention cannot but affect the experiments
she performs.

Her scientific ethic is reverence for life. Reverence for the lives
she has brought forth, the lives she aids with her science, the
lives of the plants that work in harmony with her.

She knows that when she heals a tiny part of the universe, she
is affecting the whole web, and she knows that if at any step of
the way her medicine harms—in its creation, in its use, or in
its elimination—it harms all.

So first . . . so first,
when women practice science, first . . . they DO NO HARM.

RECIPES FOR FRESH LEAVES, HEMP SEEDS, AND HEMP SEED OIL

Hemp seed oil is usually labeled as hemp oil and found in the refrigerated section of the health food store. Although it loses some of its essential fatty-acid superpowers when heated, it will help pull the medicine out of your tea.

Warning: Do not confuse hemp seed oil with concentrated cannabis medicines that are often confusingly called "hemp oil."

✹ Herbal Pesto

Makes about 1 cup

Ingredients

4 cups gently packed cannabis leaves, chopped small

2 cups gently packed herb leaves, chopped small (lemon balm, dandelion, cilantro, basil, arugula, etc.)

½ cup hemp seeds or any other nuts

2 garlic cloves chopped small

¼ teaspoon salt, pepper to taste

½ cup hemp oil or any other tasty oil (I like to blend hemp and olive oil)

½ cup grated parmesan cheese or any other hard cheese (optional)

1. Combine half of the leaves with the nuts, garlic, cloves, salt, and a little oil in a blender or food processor. Blend continuously until the ingredients are finely chopped. Use a blender for a smoother paste or food processor for a chunkier dip.

2. Scrape down the sides of the bowl and add the rest of the leaves. Blend until a uniform paste has formed. Scrape down the sides of the bowl as needed.

3. With the blender running, stream in the oil. Less oil will make a paste good for spreading on sandwiches and pizzas; more oil will make a sauce better for pastas and stirring into soup. Scrape down the sides of the bowl

and continue blending as needed until the oil is emulsified into the leaves and the pesto looks uniform.

4. Taste the pesto and add more salt, garlic, nuts, or cheese as needed to taste.

5. Storing: Pesto will darken and brown very quickly, but will still be tasty and fresh for several days. For best appearance, use it right away. If storing, store it in the smallest container possible and thoroughly press the pesto to eliminate air pockets. Pour a little oil or lemon juice over the surface, cover, and refrigerate for up to a week. Pesto can also be frozen for several months, but it is better to freeze it without the cheese in it. Add the cheese after thawing. Freeze in single serving sizes.

Warning: Raw cannabis leaves can become psychoactive if exposed to heat. Make sure the blender does not get too hot or you do not put the pesto on very hot food if you don't want this effect.

🌿 Green Goddess Dressing

Ingredients

2 tablespoons chopped fresh cannabis leaf

2 tablespoons chopped fresh lemon balm, thyme, spearmint, basil, oregano, or fresh herb of your choice

2 calendula blossoms, fresh or dried

2 tablespoons dried nettles, crumbled

6 tablespoons hemp oil

4 tablespoons olive oil

2 tablespoons apple cider vinegar

1 tablespoon fresh lemon juice

2 cloves minced garlic

Salt and freshly ground pepper to taste

Blend ingredients in a blender until smooth. Add more oil if needed.

Warning: Raw cannabis leaves can become psychoactive if exposed to heat. Make sure the blender does not get too hot or you do not put the dressing on very hot food if you don't want this effect.

🌿 Sinsemilla Salsa

Ingredients

2 cups plum tomatoes, diced

¼ cup chopped white onion

3 tablespoons chopped fresh cannabis leaf

3 tablespoons chopped fresh cilantro

2 teaspoons minced jalapeño (remove seeds for less heat)

1½ teaspoons fresh lime juice

1 small garlic clove, minced

Salt to taste

Toss all ingredients together until well combined.

Warning: Cannabis leaves can become psychoactive if exposed to heat. Do not cook salsa or blend into hot food if you want to avoid this effect.

🌿 Hemp Tabbouleh

I recommend this medicinal delicious salad for most of my clients. It's packed full of protein and essential fatty acids as well as medicine from the fresh herbs. It is ideal for those who can only manage a few bites of food. It can be eaten as a salad or sprinkled on just about anything.

Ingredients

2 cups raw shelled hemp seed

3 tablespoons hemp oil

3 tablespoons sunflower oil

3 tablespoons fresh lemon juice

1–3 tablespoons soy sauce or Bragg's Amino Acids to taste

½ cup finely chopped fresh cannabis leaf

½ cup finely chopped herbs (more cannabis leaf, parsley, dandelion leaf, calendula petals, lemon balm leaf, mint, chickweed, arugula, etc.)

Optional Ingredients

½ cup sliced black olives

½ cucumber, diced, no seeds

Toss all ingredients together until well combined.

DIY GANGA TEAS

A cup of tea is a cup of humanity, delighting the soul and strengthening the will. Perhaps the most common ritual in the world is serving a cup of tea, and perhaps hemp was the first tea and the first tea ritual.

We make teas from dried plants, fresh plants, or a combination. We make them from leaves, flowers, bark, berries, roots, and fruits, with water, milk, or fruit juice. There are as many ways to enjoy this ritual as there are leaves in a pot.

Recipes for preparing teas usually call for one (or more) of the following methods:

Steeping and Cold Infusion: Steeping means soaking herbs in hot water. Put a lid on the cup or pot to retain the essential oils in the herbs that would otherwise evaporate away in the steam. When the tea is ready, lift the lid and allow the condensation there to drip back into the tea. Tea can be infused using hot liquid (steeping) or by cold infusion. Cold water infusions usually need 4–24 hours to reach their full strength. Steeping and infusions are usually used for the leaves, needles, and flowers of plants.

Decocting and Infusing: We decoct teas by simmering herbs in a pot with a lid over low heat. We can further reduce a decoction by removing the lid to allow water to evaporate away, thus making a stronger tea. Decocting is often necessary to infuse dried berries, roots, and "tough" leaves and seeds. It is the first step to making a syrup and also a good method for making cannabis root tea.

Sometimes a tea contains decoctions and infusions, especially when it contains dried roots and fresh flowers or leaves. In some of my recipes I make a decoction, then turn off the heat, sprinkle in leaves, place a lid on the pot, and allow it to steep for five minutes before straining.

Consumed for eons, and still used by Jamaican mothers to keep their families healthy (see "The Reproductive System," chapter 5), the little-known ganja teas are a lovely way to take your medicine, enjoy some quiet time, or complete a meal. They are a great introduction to marijuana medicine for those who are nervous about using marijuana for the first time. The medicine will target the digestive system and continue into the blood system through the liver. The onset of effect will be between 20 minutes and 1.5 hours depending on whether it is taken on an empty stomach and the digestive processing time of the tea drinker.

Leaves and flowers merely need steeping. Roots need to be ground up and simmered for 5–10 minutes. Since cannabinoids and essential oils and terpenes are fat-soluble, to make a stronger tea we add fat, like hemp seed oil, milk, coconut oil, butter, or ghee (clarified butter).

Whenever making a hot tea, steep or simmer the tea with a lid on so that the aromatic and medicinal essential oil and terpenes are not lost to evaporation. Lift the lid when the tea is no longer steaming, and pour the condensation inside the lid back into the tea.

As with most herbal medicines, Mary Jane works and tastes better when blended with her herbal friends. Simply adding some marijuana leaves to your favorite tea blend is an excellent way to begin exploring the world of marijuana teas.

Non-psychoactive Weed Teas

Non-psychoactive teas are excellent for children, elders, and pets. They make a great introduction to cannabis medicine. They still carry ganja's other medicinal properties. Psychoactive teas affect us sooner than edibles because we absorb them faster. Both can be added to other teas, so put the kettle on and sift together your favorite blend.

If you are using cannabis roots, weed with little to no THC, or are making cold infusions or sun tea, you can experiment at will in finding your favorite recipes without concern about activating THC to its psychoactive temperature. Since cannabinoids and essential oils and terpenes are fat-soluble, to make a stronger infusion we add fat or oil, like hemp seed oil, milk, coconut oil, butter, or ghee.

✹ Root Tea

Simmer 10–20 g of fresh or dried cannabis roots, chopped small or ground in a coffee grinder, per cup of water for 10 minutes in a covered pot.

Filter and enjoy hot or cold.

May be blended with any food or beverage.

✹ Fresh Leaf Tea

Fill a pint-sized mason jar ¾ full with fresh whole pot leaves and water.

Add 2 fresh buds for stronger tea, and for even stronger tea add a fat.

Put the lid on, shake well, and leave the jar in the sun for 1–3 hours.

Filter and serve cold or at room temperature.

May be blended with other cold teas and drinks.

Further Options for Fresh Leaf Tea

CBD: Choose ganja leaves that are high in CBD and very low in THC—like a 20:1 ratio or higher. May be blended with other teas or in soup.

Hot Combo: Combine CBD leaves and roots to make a whole-plant cuppa!

Cool Combo: Combine fresh or dried CBD leaves with fresh THC leaves and your premade root tea. Cover and leave in the sun for an hour. Filter and serve chilled or at room temperature.

Psychoactive Teas

When we want some of the spiritual or psychoactive effects of THC weed, we need to make hot tea. For a stronger effect, since cannabinoids and essential oils are fat-soluble, add a fat or oil like hemp seed oil, milk, coconut oil, or ghee. THC-rich tea can offer a strong psychospiritual-activating effect, depending on how strong you make it, because when THC passes through the liver it is processed into metabolites that are five to ten times stronger than THC itself. If you are concerned about overmedicating with THC, keep some CBD medicine handy as an antidote, or drink some lemonade and eat some black pepper, the ancient antidotes!

🌿 Super Psychoactive Ganja Tea

Put 1–2 grams of ground ganga bud and 2 teaspoons of hemp seed oil, milk, coconut oil or ghee per cup of water into a pot. Simmer with a lid on for 5 minutes. Filter and enjoy. May be blended with any other tea or soup. Initial dose depends on your tolerance level for THC. If you are new to THC, start with a few sips and wait for 2 hours to evaluate the effect.

TINCTURES AND LINIMENTS

Tinctures are one of the most ancient ways to concentrate and preserve plant medicine. People began making herbal tinctures using beer and wine. Cannabis-infused wine was used in ancient China as an anesthetic and analgesic. When humans learned to distill their wine into a higher proof alcohol, they not only drank it but also used it to make medicine. Since alcohol absorbs through the skin, alcohol tinctures can also be applied topically; in which case, they are called liniments.

Psychoactivity of Tinctures

It's important to understand how to control the psychoactivity of a cannabis tincture. Since traditional tinctures are made without heat, they remain relatively non-psychoactive whether using fresh and/or dried cannabis. It is hard to judge the psychoactivity of purchased tinctures, as they may have been decarboxylated (making the THC active) purposefully or even accidentally. The THCA content (the precursor for THC) may have been accurately reported on the label at the time of bottling, but some of that THCA could have converted to THC just from sitting on a sunny shelf too long or being shipped during a heat wave. Another reason for making your own!

To make a tincture with little to no psychoactivity, you can use fresh cannabis, dried or fresh root, dried leaf or a small amount of dried flower that has not been decarboxylated, a low-THC/high-CBD cannabis, or a combination of these. It's always good to add a few buds or leaves that have not been "decarbed" so that you have a more whole medicine with a wider variety of cannabinoids and terpenes. To increase the THC effects of the tincture, decarboxylate leaves and flowers before putting them into the alcohol.

How to Decarboxylate Weed

To decarboxylate your leaves and flowers and activate the THC, lay your leaves and/or buds in a single layer in a baking dish with a lid to capture the terpenes and essential oils. (You can create a lid with tin foil, but line it with parchment paper so the foil does not touch the bud and contaminate it with aluminum.) Heat the weed in the oven for an hour at 250 degrees F.

Menstruums for Tinctures

Alcohol

My preferred menstruum for cannabis tincture is alcohol. It is the strongest extraction solvent used in tincture making and has a shelf life of more or less forever. To ensure an indefinite shelf life for your medicine as well, use at least 40 percent (80 proof) alcohol. The other 60 percent is water, which is also an excellent menstruum for plant chemicals. Alcohols higher than 100 proof (like Everclear or Bacardi 151) are too strong for a basic cannabis tincture because they extract all of the fats and waxes in the plant material as well, making a very sticky tincture that adheres to the glass bottle and applicators. Be aware that whiskey, brandy, tequila, and other common alcohols usually contain artificial (toxic) colors and flavors—and they do not have to list ingredients on their labels. Organic vodka or gin are my favorites when I can find them, but I come from a medicine-making tradition that has used brandy for hundreds of years.

Glycerin

Glycerin is a traditionally used menstruum in the herbal world, but it does not extract well from cannabis leaf or flower. Glycerin extracts sugars, water-soluble proteins, and mucilaginous substances and will act as a preservative. It is actually great for cannabis roots, but it is not generally able to dissolve the fats, oils, resins, or terpenoids in the leaves and flowers. If you are tincturing the whole plant, just add some glycerin to the alcohol, or you can make a root tincture separately using glycerin, and then blend it into an alcohol tincture of the leaves and flowers.

Vinegar

Vinegar is another traditionally used menstruum in the herbal world. It is usually used for extracting alkaloids, vitamins, and minerals. It is a good menstruum for the roots and seeds of cannabis, because that is where those things are located. Because vinegar is acidic, it is not an effective menstruum for plant acids like the cannabinoid acids found in fresh cannabis. There is no research on its ability to extract cannabinoids, but I think it would be low.

Tips for Tinctures

When working with fresh herbs only, I make what are called *simpler's tinctures.* I wilt the herb overnight, and then I fill a jar with the herb and add the alcohol. To prevent oxidation, I don't leave a lot of air space between the liquid and the lid, instead filling the jar to cover the plant material.

When working with dried herbs, which are more potent (they are not diluted with water like fresh herbs), I use a ratio of 1 part herb to 5 parts alcohol. If I have 2 ounces of herb, I use 10 ounces of alcohol.

For the most part, I tincture individual herbs separately, then blend the tinctures into a formula. However, with common formulas, I might blend five herbs together first, then add the alcohol and tincture them all together. (Formulating can be a rather advanced skill, so if you are a beginner, stick to single-herb tinctures.)

It is perfectly OK to mix dried and fresh herbs together in your tincture. In the case of cannabis, the fresh herb holds completely different medicine than the dried herb, so a holistic medicine would contain both. Since fresh cannabis is available at a different time of year than the roots, I might tincture them separately and blend the finished tinctures together later.

Include the whole plant. A holistic tincture includes as many parts of a plant as possible. For cannabis specifically, this also includes fresh, dried, and decarboxylated (heated) leaves, and flowers. Roots do not need to be decarboxylated (as far as we know), so I just add some chopped or powdered root—both fresh and dried if possible.

When the tincture is ready, cap and label your jar of tincture with the name and condition of the plants, the menstruum used, and the date. You might want to include the phase of the moon, your mood, astrological events, and so on. Leave the jar in a cool, dark place for 4–6 weeks. Strain out the plant matter and you have a very powerful medicine!

If you are like many folks and only have access to dried flowers (buds), or you are not interested in the spiritual booster, just drop your buds into a jar, add enough alcohol to cover the buds, cap, and let sit for 24 hours to 6 weeks. Presto, you've made your first cannabis tincture!

🜀 Basic Holistic Cannabis Tincture Recipe

Clean and smudge your work area.

Wilt 1 ounce of fresh leaves and 2 fresh flowers overnight.

Chop them small and put them in a small glass jar.

Add 1 ounce of dried leaf and 1 dried bud, chopped small.

Add ½ ounce of dried root, powdered or chopped small.

While you are handling your herbs, take a minute to offer thanks and to ask them to infuse your medicine with healing power.

Take enough vodka to almost fill the jar, minus ¼ cup. Blend in ¼ cup of vegetable glycerin.

Use the extra ¼ cup of vodka to make yourself a cocktail.

Pour your blended menstruum over the herb to the top of the jar.

Put on the lid and give it a gentle shake.

Put in your intentions for the medicine.

Label the jar with the contents and date.

Utilize any knowledge of astrology, crystals, minerals, or other healing modalities to strengthen your medicine.

Store in a cool, dark place for 4–6 weeks.

Note: Although we leave the tincture to fully infuse for 4–6 weeks, you can actually start using the medicine after 24 hours, it just won't be as strong.

Strain tincture.

Although not necessary, you may then choose to filter the tincture through several layers of cheesecloth, filter paper, or muslin.

Be the first to try your medicine. Begin with a small dose, maybe 5 drops in water or under the tongue. Evaluate, and increase the dose until you realize its power.

Then offer it to friends in exchange for feedback. You can now blend this tincture with others in a formula if you want.

Store in a cool, dark place.

INFUSED OILS

Infusing herbs into oil creates a magical medicine that can be used internally or topically. Ancient desert tribes rubbed in plant oils to wash themselves instead of using ever-scarce water. Socrates praised olive oil as the "assuager of pain." Plant-infused oils are often confusingly called herbal oils, medicinal oils, or infused oils.

> *Warning:* Do not confuse infused oils with essential oils, which are a distilled concentrate, or with a concentrated cannabis medicine often called "CBD oil," "hemp oil," or sometimes just "oil."

Oils will extract most fatty acids, fixed oils, lipids, waxes, steroids, triterpenoids, steroidal alkaloids, gums, resins, and oleoresins from the plants used. They will partially extract alkaloids, essential oils, mucilage, allantoin, and hypericins. Agricultural pesticides are also soluble in oil, so use only organic ingredients and oils.

Infused oils are nutritive and good for pain relief, inflammation, skin conditions, moisturizer, skin protection, lubricants, and for beauty treatments. They are also ideal bases for salves and lotions.

Which Oils to Choose

Your choice of oils is dependent on whether your infused oil is for internal or external use. Regardless of your choice, always use the highest quality organic vegetable oils possible for medicine making. I often use olive oil or coconut oil, as both can be used internally or externally and are very nutritive either way. Other commonly used oils include sesame, almond, grape-seed, or jojoba.

Olive oil is extremely rich in monounsaturated fats and antioxidants. It has strong anti-inflammatory, anticancer, and antibacterial properties. Its consumption has been shown to prevent strokes and heart disease and relieve arthritis. It can help prevent and remove plaque buildup in the brain that causes dementia and Alzheimer's disease. Topically, it moisturizes skin and protects it from bacterial growth and oxidative damage. Use extra virgin olive oil because it is less refined than the other grades and retains the most antioxidants and bioactive compounds from the olives.

Coconut oil is rich in a unique combination of fatty acids called medium-chain triglycerides (MCTs) that kill harmful pathogens like bacteria, viruses, yeast, and funguses. It is effective against antibiotic-resistant staph infections like MRSA, caused by the bacterium *Staphylococcus aureus*. It is also effective against the yeast *Candida albicans,* a common source of yeast infections. It been shown to improve brain function, boost metabolism (resulting in weight loss), and help epileptic patients by contributing to a ketogenic diet that seems to reduce seizures. A diet rich in coconut oil also improves insulin sensitivity and reduces the risk of type 2 diabetes. Because medium-chain triglycerides bypass the stomach and go directly to the liver, coconut oil infused with cannabis and other herbs will act faster and have an increased bioavailability. Coconut oil is anti-inflammatory and analgesic whether applied topically or ingested.

Topically, coconut oil moisturizes the skin and can reduce symptoms of eczema. It provides weak protection from the sun, blocking about 20 percent of the sun's ultraviolet rays. Used in the mouth, it kills harmful bacteria and improves dental health.

There are many other rich and nutritious vegetable oils that can be used alone or blended for herbal infusions, like the above-mentioned sesame, almond, grape-seed, or jojoba oil. Jojoba oil is closest to the oils naturally produced by our skin. And, of course, there is hemp seed oil, one of the most nutritious and medicinal oils known. However, hemp seed oil is too delicate to heat, so I often blend it into a formula after the herbs have been infused.

How to Infuse Oils

An infused oil is made by steeping dried or fresh herbs in vegetable oil with gentle heat for a period of time that's specific to the heat source. Chemical constituents are "digested" from the herbs into the oil. The herbs are then filtered out and pressed. The now-infused oil is filtered and ready for external, and sometimes internal, use.

Dried herbs or fresh? Dried herbs are easier to infuse for the simple reason that the water in fresh herbs doesn't mix well with oil and can provide a substrate for bacteria that leads to rotting herbs. However, fresh cannabis is wonderfully medicinal, and many other herbs are best infused when they are fresh. When using fresh herbs in an infusion, wilt the herbs overnight to remove excess water, and leave the lid of the infusing vessel open to allow water to evaporate out of the infusion. Once again, you can infuse herbs singly or formulate a blend and infuse them together.

Solar as Heat Source

The most traditional and sustainable heat source is the sun, which can provide the preferred target temperature range of 100–120 degrees F. I place my containers in direct sun. Some worry that direct sun will break down the oil. Although that has never happened to me, probably due to the preservative effects of the herbs and my personal spiritual relationship with the sun, if you prefer, you can also put the jar in a paper bag before leaving it in the sun. Check the temperature of your infusion regularly—I cannot leave mine in the hot summer sun at my home, because it will heat to over 120 degrees F. Since the infusion cools down at night, it needs 2–4 weeks to ensure "full digestion."

Woodstove or Heater as Heat Source

In the winter, I place my infusing oils by the woodstove for 4–6 weeks. My woodstove is hot during the day and cold at night so this method takes 4–6 weeks. Check the temperature regularly to avoid overcooking. Try for the optimum range of 100–120 degrees F.

Crockpot as Heat Source

If your heat source is continuous, you only need to infuse your herbal oil for a week. In the summer I use a crockpot. Put your jar of herbs covered with oil in a water bath in a crockpot with the temperature set for 100 to 120 degrees F for a week. Leave a loose lid on the jar to allow any moisture to escape but prevent dust from getting in. Alternatively, you can place your herbs directly into the crock and completely cover them with oil. Put a lid on the crock, and set the temperature between 100 and 120 degrees F for a week. These should not be left unattended, of course, but will not burn at that low of a temperature.

Be careful, because most crockpots get too hot above 120 degrees F, even on the warm setting. You can test your crockpot temperature by filling it with water, leaving it on the lowest setting overnight, and then checking the temperature of the water. If it is too hot, it can be modified by adding a dimmer switch to the crockpot's cord.

Slow Oven Method

Place your herbs and oil in a canning jar. Place the canning jar in a large water bath so that the water reaches a quarter of the way up the jar. Place in the oven at 110–120 degrees F for one week. This is safe for electric or gas ovens because the temperature is so low. If you want a very psychoactive oil, decarboxylate the weed first.

Warning: Always put jars in a water bath so they don't break! The bath will capture spilled oil if they do. If a jar breaks and oil spills in the oven this can cause a grease fire. Turn off the oven immediately. Do not put water on a grease fire. Use salt or a fire extinguisher.

Quick Oven Method

Follow directions for the Slow Oven Method, but instead of 1 week at a low temperature, infuse the oil at 250 degrees F for 1–2 hours. Due to the high heat needed to decarboxylate the pot and infuse the oil quickly, for this method I prefer to use coconut oil, because it has a high tolerance for heat. (Olive oil might oxidate/cook at this temperature.)

Whatever your method, remember to crack the lids if you are infusing fresh herbs, and check the jars regularly for pokeys. Smell and taste the oil as it is infusing so you get to know it and develop an instinct for when it is "done."

Straining and Filtering

To strain out the herb, pour the herb-oil mixture through a sprouting screen, a strainer, or a funnel lined with a piece of cheesecloth or muslin that is large enough to catch a handful of the herb. Clean cotton handkerchiefs or T-shirt material also work well. Squeeze out the herb in the cloth or use a salad spinner (which I call a "poor girl's centrifuge") to remove excess oil from the plant matter. You can then use the cloth full of oily herb to rub on your skin or put in the bath.

It's best to allow the crude oil to settle overnight so plant matter and any water will settle at the bottom. You can then decant the oil through another filter of several layers of cheesecloth or muslin.

> *Warning:* Do not discard oily THC cannabis outdoors or in your compost pile, as animals love it, and they can knock themselves out for a few days if they get into it!

Storing

Store in an airtight container in a cool, dark place.

An infrequently opened container can have a shelf life of 1–5 years, depending on the herb used, so pour out small amounts into a smaller bottle for daily use. Do not put dirty spoons or fingers into the oil. You can extend the shelf life by adding natural preservatives like rosemary extract, vitamin E, and/or essential oils.

You will know if your infused oil has gone bad from the rancid smell or if mold appears. Do not worry if your medicines go bad. It happens to everyone. Give them back to the Earth where animals can't get at them, and try again!

✳ Solar-Infused Whole Plant Cannabis Infused Oil

Ingredients

1 cup fresh cannabis leaf and flower, chopped finely

1 cup decarboxylated leaf and flower, crumbled or ground

½ cup dried root, powdered

½ cup fresh root, chopped as small as possible

4 cups olive oil

4 cups coconut oil

Spread all fresh herb out on a tray to wilt overnight.

Blend the coconut and olive oils together.

Loosely pack your herbs into a clean, dry quart-sized mason jar. They should fill between ½ and ¾ of the jar. Be sure to leave a minimum of 2–3 inches at the top of the jar.

Pour in enough oil to cover the herbs by at least 1 inch. Mix very gently with a chopstick to avoid plant matter sticking to the sides of the jar that are above the liquid. If this happens, wipe excess away with a paper towel.

Put the lid on the jar and let sit overnight. Add more oil in the morning if it is no longer covering the herbs by 1 inch.

Be very careful that there are no "pokeys." If any of the plant matter is breaking the surface of the oil, it can introduce bacteria and rot.

When infusing fresh herbs, leave the lid cracked to allow water to evaporate out.

Place the jar in a brown paper bag, with the lid cracked, and leave in a sunny place for 2–4 weeks. You do not want the formula heated above 120 degrees F, so if you are in a hot climate, move the jar to the shade for the hottest part of the day. Check the oil daily with a thermometer, by smelling it, and by tasting it. Use a clean utensil, not your finger!

When you feel the infusion is ready, place a large piece of cheese cloth or a sprouting screen over the jar opening and secure with a lid ring. Invert the bottle to strain the oil into a container, preferable one with a pour spout.

Remove the ring and place the plant matter in cheesecloth or a piece of muslin and squeeze the excess oil from the plant matter. You can also use a salad spinner to remove the excess oil from the plant matter.

Let the crude oil settle overnight to allow plant matter and any water to settle at the bottom of the jar. You can then decant the oil through another filter of several layers of cheesecloth or muslin.

Store in an airtight container in a cool, dark place. Infused oils have a limited shelf life of 1–5 years, depending on the herbs used and how often you open the container. You may want to store in several small containers. You will know when they go bad from the smell or if mold appears.

☘ Basic Slow Infusion Oil Recipe

Pack a mason jar to within 2–3 inches of the top with your chopped, ground, or crumbled herb or herbs.

Pour in enough oil cover the herb by at least 1 inch. Let sit overnight. Top off oil in the morning. When using dried herbs, you will probably have to add more oil in the morning. Be very careful at this step that there are no "pokeys." If any of the plant matter is breaking the surface of the oil, it can introduce bacteria and rot.

Put on lid loosely. The oil will expand as it warms. When infusing fresh herbs, I leave the lid cracked to allow water to evaporate out.

Keep infusion between 100 and 120 degrees F for about 1 week. Check aroma and flavor daily.

☘ Quick Oven Recipe for Cannabis-Infused Coconut Oil

Preheat oven to 280 degrees F.

Warm ½ gallon of coconut oil to a liquid state. A glass jar of coconut oil with the lid loosened can be placed in the oven in a water bath while the oven heats.

Fill another ½ gallon canning jar with 100–150 g of cannabis leaf and crumbled buds (and some chopped dried root if available!) to up to 2 inches below the shoulders of the jar.

Pour liquid coconut oil over the herb until it covers the cannabis by ½ inch.

Put the jar into a water bath pan with the water reaching ¼ of the way up the jar. Canning jars are designed to take a water bath. Do not try to heat them dry or they might crack. (The water bath will also capture spilled oil if they do break, thus reducing risk of an oven grease fire or just a huge mess!)

Put the jar in the oven for an hour. The contents will reach 240–265 degrees F, thus decarboxylating the cannabinoids and also infusing them into the oil.

Remove the jar and place a sprouting screen or cheese cloth over the opening and secure it with a lid ring. Invert the bottle to strain the oil.

Fine filter the oil using cheese cloth. Remaining sediment will fall to the bottom of the jar.

SALVES

❋ Basic Recipe

Warm any vegetable oil or infused vegetable oil in a double boiler.*

Melt in shredded beeswax, beeswax pastilles, or another hard fat like cocoa butter until the desired consistency is reached. I start with a cupped handful of beeswax per cup of oil. An exact measurement would be 17 grams of wax per 100 ml of oil.

To test consistency, drop a drop on your arm and wait until it cools. You can also place a spoon in the freezer for five minutes and then dip your frozen spoon in the mixture.

A harder consistency is desired for salves that you don't want to melt easily, like lip balms. A softer consistency is better for salves that will be rubbed in, like a salve for sore muscles or joints.

---

*To make your own double boiler, place stones or the rings from mason jars in the bottom of a pot. Place a Pyrex measuring cup on top so that the bottom of the cup does not touch the bottom of the pot. Add water to the pot until it reaches halfway up the cup. Take care that boiling water does not jump into your oil.

AROMATHERAPY MEDICINES USING
ESSENTIAL OILS AND HYDROSOLS

Aromatherapy blends are great remedies because you can carry them with you and use at the first sign of anxiety, exposure to infectious disease, depression, and so on. Their aromas encourage deep breathing and bring a sense of calm and well-being. I've seen these work wonders for clients, and I have successfully introduced them to many harried mothers with crying babies on airplanes or in restaurants. Both the mothers and the babies calm right down! Both hydrosols (flower waters) and essential oils can be used for aromatherapy, as well as pieces of your favorite aromatic plant.

✹ Spritzers to Dispense Aromas

Fill a 4-ounce spray bottle with 1.5 ounces of distilled water and 1.5 ounces of alcohol. (This leaves plenty of space in the bottle so you can shake the bottle well before each use.)

Add 3 drops of Rescue Remedy or other desired flower essence.

Add 30–40 drops of the essential oil(s) of your choice. Essential oils vary in strength and change with time, so be prepared to adjust the recipe the next day after it has had time to blend.

Always shake well before spraying.

✹ Topical Oils

Add 10–12 drops of essential oils per ounce of carrier oil for massage, foot soaks, handkerchiefs, or rollerballs.

✹ Steams

Blend a few drops of essential oil, depending on how strong the oil is, into a carrier oil. Float a few drops of the oil blend in a bowl of steaming water. Close your eyes, bend your face over the bowl, and place a towel over your head and the bowl. Inhale gently and allow the steam to bathe your face. Or you can add the carrier oil to a steam bath or a sauna. For safety, if you are unfamiliar with the strength of the essential oil you want to use, consult an herbalist first.

✳ Soaks

Blend a few drops of essential oil, depending on how strong the oil is, into a carrier oil. Add the blend to a foot soak, hand soak, or hot bath. You can also dip a towel in and wrap it around an arm or leg. For safety, if you are unfamiliar with the strength of the essential oil you want to use, consult an herbalist first.

✳ Smudges

Light a piece of your herb or a smudge stick on fire. Blow out the flame. Set it in an ashtray and allow it to smolder. Inhale the smoke or use it to purify a room.[1] Do not leave unattended while burning.

10

The Spirit of Ganja
around the World

Hemp is woven more tightly into the fabric of humanity than any other plant. We know that cultures throughout world history have used cannabis for food, fiber, and medicine for millennia, but many also use hemp in their spiritual practices—and for an equally long time. Few of today's Christians are aware that Jesus used cannabis, and few Jews are aware that Moses did too. Buddhists have forgotten that the Buddha used cannabis, and not many Muslims are aware that cannabis is entangled in their Zoroastrian roots. Hinduism, Daoism, and many other religions and spiritualities were founded around cannabis, and thousands of shamanistic cultures throughout Africa, Asia, Europe, and the Americas developed around this magical, mystical plant.

In fact, the history of cannabis is also the history of all of humankind and all religions!

So, to truly understand Mary Jane's full power as the Queen of Herbs, we must get to know her powers in the spiritual realm as well as the physical and mental realms. We live in a world out of balance that is crying out for help, and it is time to rediscover pot's spiritual gifts and then share what we know—even in the face of stereotypes, resistance, fear, and ignorance. Be the agent of that which you love in the world.

It is in this spirit that I offer this chapter exploring the secret, sacred world of ganja. In it, I dive into myths and mystery and let stories replace science. I offer you tales that tempt faith and sorcery that seduces belief. Nothing that I write here is true, and all of it is true.

The spirit of marijuana is best experienced for yourself.

In ancient history we discover the seeds of the great religions, and together we can travel a wild path that leads to those who are currently dancing, praying, and meditating with cannabis as their guru. I will introduce ritual and prayer from different ages, mystics, tribes, and religions with a look, at the end of the chapter, at gentle ways you can experiment with bringing cannabis into your own spiritual practice. Are you ready to meet the spirit of cannabis herself?

She is sensitive, dynamic, and analytical. She learns, remembers, and can plan for the future. She creates language to communicate with herself and others and is interdependent with her community. She passes her knowledge on to others in her community—and even to future generations. She makes tools, stores them outside of herself, and uses them to adjust her surroundings.

Sensitive to changes in her environment, she registers alterations in temperature, moisture, elements in the soil, the approach of predators, and more. She can feel all that touches her and determine its nature—a raindrop? a caterpillar? her favorite cat! She perceives damage to herself and prepares defenses in response. She is self-aware and recognizes that she is separate from other organisms.

She carefully analyzes incoming data from her own neural network *and* from her environment. From this she musters potential responses. She can decide to change her shape, the chemicals she emits, and the insects she invites in or repels. She decides the location, direction, and rate of her growth, whether to reproduce or not, and the nutrients she absorbs. She can even modify the very genes in her cells.

She performs complex cost-benefit assessments so she can choose and implement the optimal course of action. With intention, she continually and successfully acclimates to her dynamic surroundings and her life. She learns. When a part of herself is cut off and planted in another place, in different soil, with different humidity, nutrients, wind, temperature, and rainfall, she will learn about her new surroundings, adapt, and thrive there.

She makes tools—impact tools—chemicals that she designs to alter her surroundings. With them she repels predators, attracts friends, pulls nutrients from the soil, and feeds the beneficial organisms in the neighborhood. She maintains storage areas outside of herself. She keeps part of her nervous system in the soil and sustains a communication network in the air around her.

She remembers her experiences by storing information in the repository of her roots. She will recall the information later, in order to make defensive and proactive decisions. She holds the acquired learning of previous generations in her genes. She passes this wisdom onto younger generations. She makes plans for the future.

Bitten by an insect, she can analyze its saliva and determine which insect it is. She can then craft a specific pheromone and release it into the air from her leaf stomata as a volatile chemical. That pheromone will call in the exact predator that eats that particular insect. Another pheromone will warn the plants around her about the danger. She can feel it when another of them is ill and will send medicine to heal it. Volatile organic compounds are her words; energetic vibrations are her sentences. They are how she communicates—with herself and her entire community. She sends and receives these messages through complicated underground mycelium highways, and through thin air. She uses the same neurotransmitters that are coursing through your body right now. She even speaks through auditory signals and clicking sounds—although in a wavelength too subtle for us to hear.

Sensing dis-ease in her grower/partner, she can produce within herself the very plant medicine needed for that person's condition. Sensing a human in danger of ignorance, she can reach out to them and instill inner wisdom.

As with all plants, she is conscious and intelligent. If you are too, then, as shamans and witches have been doing for eons, you can learn to communicate with her! Let us begin with a story . . .

THE GREAT LEAP FORWARD

This is the story of Toba, an ancient volcano that blew its top in a far-away land we now call Sumatra some seventy-five thousand years ago, when there were only one million *Homo sapiens* and Neanderthals wandering throughout today's Asian and African continents.

Although Toba had flared and flowed twice before in previous millennia, the third blast was the largest volcanic eruption on Earth in two million years. Toba had been collecting molten magma beneath the surface of the Earth for eons until one day it finally, dramatically ruptured, spewing over seven hundred cubic miles of magma and covering all of South Asia with ash fifteen centimeters thick. Ash blanketed the Indian Ocean, the Arabian Sea, and the South China Sea. Six billion tons of sulfur dioxide forced its way into the highest layer of the atmosphere and quickly spread across the world. These thick gases reflected the light and heat of the sun back into space. After fifty thousand years of stable warmth, Earth's temperature plummeted 25 degrees F, triggering a fifteen-year winter followed by an ice age that lasted for a thousand years.

Plant and animal populations crashed. And the prehumans decreased from one million to a mere ten thousand, with only between one thousand and five thousand breeding females among them. Scientists today call this a population bottleneck.

But the fascinating part of the story is what happened next: a rapid, magical era of human evolution called the "Great Leap Forward."

The "cave people" who survived began a rapid evolution in human advancement. They began making tools and art. They crafted fishhooks from bone and spear handles from wood. They began fashioning musical instruments and jewelry, painting stories on cave walls, and firing pottery. They built boats and began to organize living spaces, hunting parties, explorations, and trade networks.

And they became spiritually conscious and began performing rituals and ceremonial burials. These protohumans leapt forward to become human in an amount of time much too short to fit any theory of Darwin's, so short that it has been referred to as the "big bang of human consciousness."

To find out what triggered it, scientists focused on one region that was out of reach of Toba's long arms of destruction. In Mossel Bay, along the southern coast of South Africa, where temperatures remained moderate and food remained prevalent, modern humans came into being.

Scientists hypothesize that what triggered the rapid development of the species at that site was the seafood.

Seafood contains high amounts of the proteins and fatty acids needed for brain development. Alpha-linolenic acid (ALA), for example, is a precursor for docosahexaenoic acid (DHA), the primary structural component of the human brain. In fact, DHA makes up nearly 70 percent of a baby's brain and 60 percent of an adult brain. This omega-3 essential fatty acid is also the main ingredient of our skin, sperm, testicles, and retinas.

But I, for one, don't think that it was solely clams and mussels that provided the triggering "brain food." ALA and other essential fatty acids are also found in very high concentrations in hemp seeds. Indeed, in hemp seeds, the ratio of ALA, an omega-3 fatty acid, to linoleic acid, an omega-6 fatty acid, is 55:25—the ideal ratio for human development.

Hemp seeds carry all twenty amino acids, including the nine essential ones that must be consumed in food. Edestin is a protein unique to hemp seeds. It has a similar structure to human blood plasma and plays an important role in strengthening the immune system and helping the body adapt to stress.

Hemp seeds also have many nutrients necessary for evolution that seafood does not contain. The calyxes of hemp seeds are covered with cannabinoids that cure disease and correct cellular dysfunction through the endocannabinoid system. The highest concentration of cellular receptors for those cannabinoids lives in the brain. Hemp has the ability to improve intelligence, to increase immunity, and to resist disease. Ganja can heal injury and disease, improve vision, increase one's sense of smell, and stimulate appetite.

But perhaps the most relevant fact to ponder is that cannabis also stimulates consciousness.

So, while a high seafood diet probably could have contributed to the Great Leap Forward, it seems likely that hemp played a major part as well by increasing human intelligence, fertility, immunity, healing, vision, and spirituality.

Or even more fascinating, is hemp poised to promote the *next* step of human evolution?

Just after the end of the volcanic winter, humans began to migrate out of Africa and into Eastern Asia, Europe, and Australia. No doubt they were carrying the sacred seeds of evolution with them.

HEMP AND THE DEVELOPMENT OF HUMAN CONSCIOUSNESS

In [man's] quest for seeds and oil, he certainly ate the sticky tops of the plant. Upon eating Hemp, the euphoric, ecstatic, and hallucinatory aspects may have introduced man to the other-worldly plane from which emerged religious beliefs, perhaps even the concept of deity. The plant became accepted as a special gift of the gods, a sacred medium for communion with the spiritual world and as such it has remained in some cultures to the present.

RICHARD EVANS SCHULTES*

Imagine, for a moment, being a primitive hunter and gatherer. Try to experience the world through your ancient senses . . .

Out gathering leaves and roots in the veld, you come across this sticky bush with a heady aroma. Nibbling on her seeds you discover a rich, oily, and tasty snack. And there are enough seeds to bring back to camp and share! Others in the tribe also like the seeds and the

---

*Richard Evans Schultes was an educator at Harvard, a prolific author, and a botanist specializing in ethnobotany and psychoactive plants. His books include *Hallucinogenic Plants* and *Man and Marijuana* as well as *Plants of the Gods: Their Sacred, Healing, and Hallucinogenic Powers* and *The Botany and Chemistry of Hallucinogens,* both coauthored with chemist Albert Hofmann, the discoverer of LSD.

tender young leaves of the plant. Soon the camp floor is littered with branches of this herb as well as dozens of others. Gathering around the fire at night, you toss some of the bits and pieces around you into the flames. You notice the different aromas that drift from the flames, and soon you can identify which herbs create pleasing smoke. These you throw in more often and move closer to the fire to better inhale the smoke.

One of these herbs even seems to improve your sense of smell, and the smoke of this herb sharpens your night vision in the dark night, improves your distance vision, and, upon sunrise, you notice that colors are brighter. When you take the smoke in before leaving to hunt, you are a more patient predator—able to remain still, silent, and focused for longer periods of time. With your enhanced senses, your hunting skills improve, and your gathering is more fruitful.

Your enhanced sense of touch puts you more in tune with the rhythms of nature around you. You seek sex more often. Your moon cycle becomes healthier, and you become pregnant more easily. You have achieved an evolutionary edge, and your tribe thrives. One day, while communicating with grunts and sign language to the other hunters, you become excited, and your first word comes out. . .

Does this seem far-fetched? Not according to ethnobotanist Terence McKenna, who wrote "No plant has been a continuous part of the human family longer than the hemp plant" and believed that psychoactive substances were the catalyst for syntactic language in Neolithic humans.[1]

One day, somewhere in Africa, someone picked up a hollow reed, leaned low into the fire, and placed one end into the sweet smoke of burning herb. She placed her mouth at the other end and drew in a breath. Suddenly she was filled with the sweet smoke of the herb separated from the harsh woodsmoke. Some other day someone learned that he could carry a small coal in a nutshell to kindle another fire. If he placed his favorite herb onto the coal, the sweet smoke would drift up and he could even carry it around! At some point someone poked a hole in a nutshell and placed a straw there. Perhaps people invented pipes to smoke pot!

When human children are born, they are fully self-absorbed and unaware that those around them are living separate lives. The first sense of individuality they develop is the realization that their mother is a separate entity. Through their teenage years, they learn that all those around them have lives separate from their own, and hopefully they even learn that their behavior affects others, just as other people's behavior affects them. Following a similar path, humans evolved to notice that there were invisible forces acting on the world around them. They became aware of an undefinable "other." In realizing this they recognized themselves as separate from others, and thus they developed the ability to self-reflect.

> In his book [*The Origin of Consciousness in the Breakdown of the Bicameral Mind*], [Julian] Jaynes claims that ancient people were not as fully conscious and self-aware as modern humans. Being unable to introspect, they experienced their own higher cognitive functioning as auditory hallucinations—the voices of gods, actually heard as in the Old Testament or the Iliad—which told a person what to do in circumstances of novelty or stress. . . . Cannabis has its own unique receptor sites in the human brain, located in the areas governing higher thinking and memory. Could it be that deep interior thought grew out of language and the use of psychoactive plants like cannabis?[2]

We all have self-reflections and dreams. We have imaginary conversations with others and ourselves, in which we excuse, defend, plead our causes, and proclaim our hopes and dreams. We daydream about our futures and examine our pasts, all in our heads. Are we talking to ourselves? Are we talking to a god? Or both? Where do our dreams and plans come from?

Were humans first introduced to the spiritual world with psychoactive substances? By watching and mimicking the animals around them, people learned which herbs, plants, and mushrooms to use for food and medicine, and they also learned which to use to induce dreams and visions.

Throughout human history we have used spiritually active agents provided by Mother Nature to connect with the divine world. We now call those substances entheogens (*en* means "inner," *theo* means "god," and *gen* means "generate"). These special plants, funguses, and other natural substances helped humans develop the religions of the world and are a pivotal part of shamanism and spirituality today. Entheogens help us "engender our inner goddess."

Marijuana has always provided a path to the spirit world. In addition to her role as an entheogen, she has also been worshiped as a deity in her own right. In fact, she is the first divine being known to have been worshiped in human history, and she is still worshiped today and forms the basis for many modern-day religions.

Entheogens connect us directly to the god within, our internal divine spark, our spirit, our soul. This connection tunes us in to our inner spiritual guide and our healing energy. There are many entheogens out there acting as sacred mediators to the divine: magic mushrooms are entheogens, as are peyote and mescaline and ayahuasca, and many other plants and mushrooms that help human beings commune with nature, the energy of the universe, and gods and goddesses of all types.

Are these entheogens conscious? Do they purposefully create intoxicating agents to help humans gain consciousness? Aren't humans who are connected with nature and reflect on themselves as a part of the web likely to act in the best interest of all who share the web?

Spirituality is a faith that comes from personally *experiencing* the divine. It is rooted in direct communion between person and deity. Many of the religions that are taught, passed down the generations, forced, or indoctrinated actively work to prevent individuals from having direct spiritual experiences and replace them with sedate rituals and entrenched doctrine. Priests, politicians, and institutions outlaw and demonize entheogens because they want to disempower, imprison, and control people, societies, and even entire civilizations. But if we search, we can still see, buried deep within sterilized religions, remnants of former entheogens in the wafting of incense, baptism with holy water, ritual sips of watered wine, and lit candles that are reminiscent of fire. We do still see entheogens in their true form in modern religious practices all over the world. They have been kept protected from those who see them as a threat to their power, because "freedom of religion" is only selectively applied. But as we shall see, the use and worship of cannabis as an entheogen remains alive and well.

So, let's follow marijuana as she shapes our history, cares for our ancestors, teaches us wisdom, and introduces us to the world of the gods.

THE ORIGIN OF THE SACRAMENT

What is the origin of the ancient cannabis plant? In truth, no one knows. However, the oldest archaeological evidence of humans' relationship with hemp goes back to the Stone Age. Rope twisted from hemp, dated to 26,900 BCE, has recently surfaced in present-day Czechoslovakia. Tools that dated to 25,000 BCE and were used for breaking down hemp stalks into fibers were found in Taiwan, along with twelve-thousand-year-old pottery decorated with hemp cord imprints. Eight-thousand-year-old Mesopotamian hemp cloth has surfaced in present-day Iran/Iraq, the cradle of civilization. What were humans capable of once they discovered hemp and the power of rope and nets?

Hemp was not only used as fiber and food in the Paleolithic era but was used ritually as well. The clearest evidence of this is in her avatar: incense. The burning of aromatic herbs and plant resins was likely the first spiritual act that humans performed. Today, incense is thought of simply as something to impart a pleasant aroma, but in most cases, ancient incense included a psychoactive, or spirit-activating, drug. The Encyclopedia Britannica confirms this: "The ceremonial use of incense in contemporary ritual is most likely a relic of the time when the psychoactive properties in incense brought the ancient worshiper into touch with supernatural forces."[3]

Incense burners, or censers, were some of the first sacred objects that human beings cast in bronze and gold. Censers have been found throughout prehistoric Egyptian tombs originating from the Fifth Dynasty (twenty-fourth to twenty-fifth century BCE), and they have been found in all the temples of the ancient world. Often symbolically decorated with cosmological themes, they were used to cleanse sanctuaries, invoke emotion, invite in deities, and divine the future. They were a way, along with the candles that came later, of moving the sacred power of fire indoors.

"The oldest evidence of spiritual ingestion of marijuana," cannabis historian Chris Bennett* told me, "are censers found in the Ukraine that date from 5,500 years ago. A well-preserved Scythian censer dated to late fourth to early third centuries BCE was uncovered in an ancient burial mound. A similar ritual artifact was discovered in a mound in the Gorny Altai [western Siberia], which confirms the hypothesis of the close cultural ties among the Scythians over great distances."[4]

In a Mesopotamian epic of a great flood, circa 1800 BCE, we meet Atrahasis the Wise, the first Savior of Mankind, who burned incense before seeking visions. In the Akkadian Empire, the first in Mesopotamia, literature from circa 2300 BCE dictates worshiping your (personal) god with the proper accompaniment of incense, and Babylonian texts of that Bronze Age era refer to "interpreting portents from incense smoke."[5]

In Sumeria, King Etana wanted a son so badly that he committed all his resources to finding the plant of birth. His story was found on cylinder seals that date from 2334 BCE. In it, Etana beseeches his god, Shamash:

> O Shamash, you have dined from my fattest sheep!
> O Netherworld, you have drunk of the blood of my
>   sacrificed lambs!
> I have honored the gods and revered the spirits,
> Dream interpreters have used up my incense,
> Gods have used up my lambs in slaughter.
> O Lord, give the command!
> Grant me the plant of birth![6]

---

*Chris Bennett has been researching the historical role of cannabis in the spiritual life of humanity for more than a quarter of a century. He is coauthor of *Green Gold the Tree of Life* and *Sex, Drugs, Violence and the Bible* and author of *Cannabis and the Soma Solution* and *Liber 420*. He has also contributed chapters on the historical role of cannabis in spiritual practices in several books.

In ancient Assyria, where modern day Iran, Iraq, Turkey, and Syria meet, priests in the seventh century BCE burned an incense called *qunubu,* an Assyrian term "that shares the same root word as cannabis."[7]

In Egypt, cuneiform tablets describing marijuana incense were discovered in an ancient library dating to circa 660 BCE. "The cuneiform descriptions of marijuana in his library and the illustrated clay tablets showing censers are considered copies of much older texts, tracing the use of cannabis as incense back to the earliest beginnings of history."[8]

King Solomon (960–925 BCE) is said to have made twenty thousand gold censers for the temple of Jerusalem alone, and seventy thousand in total. The Hebrew scriptures (Old Testament) called the temple incense *kaneh.* People traded kaneh throughout the Judaic world in the form of balls of resin, or what we call hashish. Merchant trading records referenced in the Hebrew scriptures state that iron, cassia, and kaneh were among the merchandise (Ezekiel 27:19, circa 590 BCE).

The ancient followers of the Hebrew goddess Asherah worshiped with hashish ritually. Sometimes referred to as the Queen of Heaven, Asherah was the consort of the Sumerian god, Anu; the Ugaritic god, El; and the Hebrew god, Yahweh. Her shamanic priestesses mixed hemp resins with myrrh, balsam, frankincense, and other perfumes. They anointed their skin with the mixture and, of course, burned it as incense.

The ancient Greeks burned so much pot that they invented a special word for it: *cannabeizen,* "cannabis incense." It was so valued by the ancient world that the last king of Babylon, Nabonidus (555–539 BCE), moved his kingdom to Taima, in the middle of the western Arabian desert, so he could control the hashish trade between southern Arabia and the Mediterranean.

Where did this hemp incense come from? The same place much of it comes from today, the Hindu Kush, a region of the Himalayas in today's Pakistan, Afghanistan, and Kashmir. The ancients carried the Queen of Herbs down from the mountains on foot and by horse and floated her down the Indus River on barges. They sold her to merchant fleets who delivered her across the Persian Gulf to Mesopotamia and down the Arabian coast and up through the Red Sea to Egypt and Phoenicia.

Cannabis was the most widely spread incense plant in Africa, Asia, Europe, and the Middle East and the oldest censers ever found contained remnants of that conduit to the divine. But she also guided the ancients down their spiritual paths in forms other than smoke, and so might guide us down ours.

THE RITUAL OF TEA

One of the oldest rituals found in all cultures is preparing tea. I have had the pleasure of participating in tea rituals around the world—from South Carolina sweet tea served iced on the veranda in the heat and humidity of a southern summer to fresh-harvested ginseng tea in a cabin in the Appalachian Mountains to British tea with scones in London and green tea served traditionally in a Japanese garden. I've also taken small shots of strong black tea served in rounds of three with the Wolof tribe of West Africa and drunk crushed mint tea cooked over a wood fire in the Saharan Desert and served by a Tuareg camel herder. The calming, pleasurable, warming, invigorating ritual of a cup of tea has lifted me out of the deepest doldrums and strengthened my will to face many a difficult task. Found in every culture, a cup of tea is like a cup of humanity.

The ritual of cannabis tea began about seven thousand years ago (and is still going strong today). The Sredny Stog culture is traced back to the Stone Age, around 4500 BCE. Based in current day Ukraine, these proto-Indo-European tribes used hemp in a variety of ways. They were the first to twist the extremely strong plant fibers together to make cords and rope. Thereby, they were the first to domesticate horses—for who can catch and ride a wild horse without strong rope? Their pottery, a recent invention, was artistically decorated with designs made from (what else?) hemp cord.

Over centuries the Sredny Stog and other similar tribes evolved into the Scythian tribes that swept out of the Eurasian steppes in every direction and trotted across Central Asia. They carried their hemp rope and the tradition of marijuana tea with them as they explored and conquered the world during the Scythian Age, between the seventh and third centuries BCE. They galloped down between the Black and Caspian Seas, through today's Russia, and up into Siberia. They trailed into Bulgaria, Iran (Persia), and, eventually, the Hindu Kush mountains of Afghanistan and India. They ruled Northern India (Kashmir) from 400 BCE to 400 CE. Everywhere, they introduced hemp for fiber and food, but were also using it as a spiritual sacrament.

IMMERSION IN SACRED SMOKE

When nomadic, the Scythian tribes developed a new method of ingestion and switched from pottery censers (awkward to carry on horseback, perhaps?) to incense-filled tents—a habit picked up by the ancient Jewish tribes, as I discuss later.

Thanks to written descriptions by Herodotus, a Greek historian, the Scythians are known to have hotboxed their tents with "Scythian fire." They fashioned small three- or six-poled tepees with felted wool covers, placed a brazier in the center, and threw hemp seeds, still covered by their sticky spirit-activating calyxes, onto it until the shelters were saturated with smoke. Climbing in, they would bathe in the incense. Sometimes they built smaller teepees and just put their heads in and inhaled!

As Herodotus described it: "Hemp grows in Scythia: it is very like flax; only that it is a much coarser and taller plant: some grows wild about the country, some is produced by cultivation: [For funerals] the Scythians, as I said, take some of this hemp-seed, and, creeping under the felt coverings, [of their tents] throw it upon the red-hot stones; immediately it smokes, and gives out such a vapour as no Grecian vapour-bath can exceed; the Scyths, delighted, howl, and shout for joy."[9]

Multiple Scythian burial mounds, many of them containing women warriors, have been unearthed complete with caches of gold and cannabis. Every Scythian burial found has contained a hemp-smoking kit, including a little charcoal brazier.[10] In 2015, in the Caucasus region, Russian archaeologists discovered exquisitely crafted solid gold bongs that contained not just cannabis but also opium poppy residue.[11] Cannabis and opium are the prime ingredients of Soma, the ancient recipe for a sacramental tea found throughout the Vedas, the oldest religious texts on Earth.

Other nomadic tribes in the region, including the Massagetae and the Thracians (ancient Greeks and Turks), used hemp in the same way. Four hundred years after Herodotus, another Greco-Roman writer, Plutarch, mentions that after their meals the Thracians threw the tops of a plant that looked like oregano into the fire. After inhaling the fumes, the people became drunk and then so tired they fell asleep. In ancient Turkmenistan and Tajikistan people ritually drank hemp beverages and other spiritual victuals from sacred drinking cups.

Scythian fire or Scythian incense, and with it the spiritual use of hemp, spread far and wide. The Hebrew scriptures tell us that the Scythians lived, traded, and made war with the ancient Hebrews for millennia. The Semites called the Scythians the *Ashkenaz*, named for their original progenitor, the great-grandson of Noah.[12] The Ashkenaz attacked Babylonia (Iraq) and sacked Palestine in the seventh century BCE, and even named a Greek city Scythopoloi. They invaded Syria and Judea around 625 BCE. They rode out from Iran into Eastern and Western Europe, Syria, and Palestine, and cantered all the way to western China and the Tarim Basin. This cannabis cult provided the seeds from which grew the Vedic religion in India and Afghanistan, Daoism in China, Hinduism in India, as well as Judaism, Zoroastrianism, and eventually even Christianity and Islam.

Today we find remnants of Scythian cannabis rituals, often associated with death, in Russia, Mongolia, Eastern Europe, India, and Asia. The people of Poland and Lithuania believe that the spirits of the dead visit their families on the night before Christmas, and so they serve *semieniatka*, a hemp seed soup.[13] Many Latvians and Ukrainians serve hemp seed soup on Three Kings Day—celebrating the Magi, the ancient Persian magician-kings who brought gifts of incense to the baby Jesus. (Those same Magi worshiped cannabis in the form of Soma, or Hoama, as I detail below.)

In Western Europe it is still common to throw hemp seeds into the fire during harvest time as an offering to the dead—a Scythian custom passed on for over 2,500 years. And there is that most famous symbol of death—the scythe-bearing Grim Reaper. The Scythians used scythes to harvest their hemp.

If there is one great web that ties together the world's religions, it is cannabis, and it was the Scythians who spun her hempen strands.

✹ Recipe for Scythian Incense

Based on an old Mongolian recipe

> **Ingredients in Equal Parts**
> female cannabis flowers
> juniper, fir, or pine needles
> thyme leaves
> spruce, fir, or pine resin

Grind leaves and flowers to a rough powder.
Roll small balls of the resin in the powder.
Toss the incense onto glowing coals.
Inhale deeply.
Offer thanks to your Scythian ancestors.

THE OLDEST RELIGION ON EARTH

The Vedic religion (*veda* means "knowledge" in Sanskrit), which is still practiced today, and an ancient Persian religion called Mazdayasna (the worship of the Lord of Wisdom) are both descended from the Scythians. These sister religions developed simultaneously, in different but adjacent cultures, around a sacrament called Soma, which was worshiped as a plant, a sacred tea, *and* a god. Recent analysis of an archaeological find, which I discuss later, indicates that hemp may have been mixed with opium poppy and ephedra to create Soma.

In the religious texts called the Vedas, Soma was dedicated to the gods Indra and Rudra (also known as Shiva). Evidence of Shiva worship circa 6000 BCE has been found in the Indus Valley. The four Vedas were the first known religious texts produced by humankind, and they form the basis from which many modern-day religions arose. In essence, they are the "old testament" of both Hinduism and Buddhism.

The *Rig Veda,* the first of the four, was composed during the Bronze Age (roughly 1700–1100 BCE) and maintained by oral tradition until it was inscribed in the early Middle Ages. Its more than two thousand hymns are dedicated almost exclusively to Soma. An example is shown on p. 227.

In both Vedic and Mazdean mythology, the gods became all-knowing and *gained their immortality* by drinking Soma. The king of the gods, Indra, favored Soma so much that it became known as "Indra's food." Just like the Hebrew and Christian god Yahweh, the Vedic gods wanted to keep access to all knowledge and immortality to themselves, so they gave the sacred and transformative Soma to Gandharva, the god of archery, for safekeeping. But Agni, the god of fire, stole Soma from the gods and gave it to the people, which is how they came to worship cannabis.

Although not compiled until 1500–500 BCE, the four Vedas contained oral history, hymns, and myths from the ancient proto-Indo-Iranian and proto-Indo-European cultures. One of the texts, the *Atharva Veda,* was the first medical text ever written and is the basis for *ayurveda* ("the science life"), an ancient system of medicine that is still practiced today all over the world, but especially in India, Sri Lanka, and Nepal.

Tribes of Scythians appeared in ancient Iran (Persia) between 2000 and 1400 BCE. Their religion, Mazdaism, was named after their main god, *Ahuru Mazda* ("Lord of Wisdom"). The religion, later called Zoroastrianism, evolved from the same Scythian source as did the Vedic religion in India. The Persian counterpart of the Vedic texts is the Avesta, and it contains many hymns dedicated to Hoama, the Persian pronunciation of Soma. In fact, Persian Scythians were called *Haomavarga,* or "Haoma-gatherers." They worshiped many gods, including Mazda and Mithra (Mitra in India). Their magician-priests were known as *magi*—as in the magi who appear in the Bible bearing gifts of incense for the birth of the Hebrew prophet Jesus of Nazareth.

Sanctify, Soma, our mind, our heart, our intellect;
and may thy worshipers delight in thy friendship, like
*   cattle in fresh pasture,*
in thine exhilaration by the sacrificial food;
for thou art mighty. . .
Like the winds violently shaking the trees, the droughts
*   of Soma have lifted me up,*
for I have often drunk of the Soma . . .
The praise of the pious has come to me like a lowing
*   cow to her beloved calf,*
for I have often drunk of the Soma . . .
Both heaven and earth are not equal to one half of me,
for I have often drunk of the Soma . . .
I am the sun, the greatest of the great, raised to the
*   firmament;*
for I have often drunk of the Soma . . .
Soma is a sage and a seer inspired by poetry.
She clothes the naked and heals all who are sick.
The lame walk, the blind see.
Soma is a sure means of attaining divine wisdom.
It releases us from anxiety. It is the sorcerer's ceremonial fire.
We have drunk Soma and become immortal;
we have attained the light, the Gods discovered.
Soma is the Elixir of Eternal Life . . .
the Source of Happiness and the Reliever of Suffering.
Soma was obtained by men on earth, through their
*   desire for the welfare of all people.*
To those who regularly use it, it begets joy and destroys
*   every anxiety.*
Soma is the God for Gods.[14]

The Mazdean religion was the dominant religion of pre-Iranian empires for more than a millennium. The Persian Empire itself covered over two million square miles and was the largest empire that has ever existed, spreading from southern Egypt in the west to Turkey in the north, through parts of Greece, Iraq (Mesopotamia), and into parts of India. Haoma temples have even been discovered in Algeria, Tunisia, and Syria.

In Persia around 1000 BCE Mazdaism morphed into Zoroastrianism, named for its founder and prophet Zoroaster. In the Roman Empire, it morphed into Mithraism, named for the god Mithra. Although few of the ancient Avestan texts still exist, we learn about the prophet Zoroaster from those that remain, like the *Yasnas* and *Gathas*. Soma was integral to Zoroaster from his very conception. "A heavenly rain brought forth Soma plants which were consumed by cows that belonged to his earthly parents. The cows gave milk which was pressed with Hemp and drunk by the prophet's parents, who later conceived him while making love for the first time."[15]

At one point, the god Hoama appeared to Zarathustra (Zoroaster's Persian name) offering a glimpse into the future—to this very day in fact: "At the proper time, at the Haoma-pressing hour, Haoma went up to Zarathustra, who was purifying the fire and chanting the Gathas. . . . 'I am, O Zarathustra, the orderly, death-averting Haoma. . . . Press me forth to drink. Praise me for strength, like the future Revitalizers too will praise me.'"[16]

In later hymns Zoroaster praises Haoma for her healing powers and her gifts of wisdom, peace, and truth: "I call down, O golden one, your intoxication and your light and your obstruction-smashing power, your talent, your healing, your furthering, your increasing, your strength in the whole body, your all-adorned wisdom . . . so that I may go forth among the living beings . . . overcoming hostilities, conquering the Lie!"[17]

There are numerous references in Zoroastrian literature to his Haoma-induced shamanic journeys, and Haoma was also part of initiation rites for new members. Later, the name *Haoma* shifted to the name *Bhanga*, and the Avesta texts refer to Bhanga as "Zoroaster's good narcotic."[18]

After initiating himself, legend has it that Zoroaster wandered the countryside for ten years, utterly failing to convert the people to his new religion. Until, that is, he offered a great king a cup of bhanga, which inspired the king to convert. It is written in the Denkird, a text derived from the Avesta, that when the king, Vishtaspa, drank the bhanga, it "led his soul to paradise and showed him the value of accepting the religion."[19]

At that point, the Persian prophet's Haoma-worshiping beliefs began to spread throughout the realm like—well, like Scythian fire! It reigned supreme until it was severely suppressed in the seventh century by the new conquerors, the Muslims. But Zoroastrianism never died. Many adherents migrated to India, where they became known as Parsees, and today there are still hundreds of thousands of Zoroastrians and Parsees in India, Iran, and Kurdistan.

Like the Vedic Soma, the Zoroastrian use of bhanga was restricted to the elite of society, and eventually it petered out entirely. This founding herb of their religion is now forgotten by modern Zoroastrians, though its ritual use sprang forth again in Hinduism.

Zoroastrianism also had considerable influence on the development of Judaic theology. In the third century, after their first exile, the Hebrews encountered and adopted many Persian and Babylonian customs, like the concepts of "paradise," and angels, and the afterlife. Were these new ideas accepted under the influence of kaneh-bosm? It seems likely.

In Europe, as worship shifted from the god Mazda to the god Mithra, Mazdaism/Zoroastrianism morphed into the Mithraic religion that continued to thrive and evolve with the divine guidance of Haoma. They often worshiped in underground caves infused with Haoma incense. At the turn of the millennium during the Roman Empire, Mithraism was dominant over the hundreds of sects of Christianity that had sprung forth since the death of Jesus. That is until the last Mithraist emperor lost the battle of Chrysopolis against Rome's Emperor Constantine. Soon after, Constantine converted to Christianity and made it the state religion, forcing everyone in the Roman Empire to convert. In this way he and the priests could better control the people. In 377 the rulers ordered the closing of Mithra temples, and Theodosius I in 394 declared the persecution of all non-Christian "cults." The ensuing persecution and elimination of pagans and of pot, herbal medicine, women healers, and wisdom, was all-encompassing, tortuous, and severe. It led to centuries of inquisitions that forced the Western world into the Dark Ages.

But you can't keep a good herb down . . .

Temples Out of Time

Many of the ancient sacred Avesta texts have been lost to the pillage and plunder of conquerors over the ages. So was the recipe for Soma/Haoma. Religious scholars, anthropologists, archaeologists, and many others have been searching for this ancient recipe and debating its contents for thousands of years. The scholars least hampered by their own conservative or religious perspectives reached the conclusion that the elixir contained entheogens, or spiritually active compounds. By the 1960s, Western anthropologists were realizing that many, if not all, shamanistic cultures partook of "magic" substances like mushrooms, cacti, funguses, vines, toad secretions, and other arcane elixirs to increase their knowledge, develop their consciousness, and commune with the spirit world. Knowledge of Soma's ingredients was a matter of debate until the 1970s, when archaeologists found exciting evidence in the mountains where Iran, Afghanistan, and Turkmenistan meet: temples dedicated solely to the worship of Soma!

Dating back to 1900 BCE, these temples provided the first material evidence corroborating the ancient hymns and stories of the Vedic and Avestan texts.[20] Likely of Scythian origin, they were constructed by a culture called the Bactria-Margiana, which was named after the oases the people lived in. Deep in the center of the temples, where presumably only the priestly class had access, archaeologists found all-white rooms with giant vats dug into the walls and floors. These chalk-lined vats still contained traces of the ancient sacrament that was created within them, and that is how we finally re-discovered the magical recipe for Soma: opium poppy, ephedra, and, of course, bhanga! And what did the discoverers see when they wandered outside the temple? Fields and fields of feral hemp, thickets of *ma huang* (ephedra), and meadows of colorful poppies.

The hymns of the Avesta and *Rig Veda* give details describing how priests processed these sacred plants into the Soma beverage. They began by steeping the plants in water. Reserving this tea, they then filtered out the plants and ground them up with milk, using huge stone pestles and mortars. Then they squeezed out the milky pulp using special pressing stones and poured the resulting liquid into self-supporting ceramic strainers covered with wool filters. The Sanskrit root for the words *Soma* or *Haoma* means "to press," "to pound," or "the thing that is squeezed."

The Avesta speaks of the "first priests of the mortar" and describes the final stage of creation in which the milky tea is blended with barley, sour milk, and water and poured into sacred vessels decorated with images of hemp, opium, and ephedra. The priests fermented this mixture for days before consuming it in ceremonies. The priests accompanied the entire ritual by singing and chanting the hymns written in the Avesta.

It is believed that the creation and consumption of Soma/Haoma was entirely in the control of the priestly class and was withheld from the people, except when provided during religious rituals. These practices served their gods well until, like all religions, the great Soma and Haoma cults began to fade away. Eventually, people became disenchanted with the mainstream Vedic religion as its excessive emphasis on overly complex rites and rituals offered little to the layperson who sought a direct connection with the divine. Eventually, as the religion shifted, Indra's favorite food was "outlawed," and the recipes were lost. Without Soma, the worship of Indra faded, and the ancient Soma and Haoma cults morphed into new religions like Hinduism in India and Zoroastrianism in Persia.

But you can't keep a good herb down . . .

THE TREE OF LIFE

Archaeologists found other fascinating and spiritually significant items in the Bactria-Margiana Soma temples. The floors of the white rooms were littered with tea-sipping straws made from fine, hollowed-out bones, and with ceramic chalices adorned with symbolic images, including eyes with dramatic, overly large pupils and the Tree of Life, another fascinating ancient symbol.

The Tree of Life is now best known from references in the Bible, but as the Tree of Life, Tree of Knowledge, and World Tree it is a widespread archetypal symbol found in shamanistic cultures, mythologies, and even symbols of state around the world. It may represent connection, immortality, attainment of knowledge, and physical and spiritual healing.

Archaeologist Diana Stein of the University of London traces the sacred tree motif back to paleolithic rock art in the Zagros Mountains of Iraq (once Mesopotamia). She proposes that "the motifs originally alluded to ritual trance experiences" and "they were adopted over the millennia during the formalization of religious practice and by rulers of the state and . . . quite possibly inspired the story of the fall of man in Genesis."[21]

Stein further believes that cannabis is the most likely candidate for the sacred tree. Depicted on countless seals and steles throughout history in that region, the sacred tree is often shown growing in the mountains. It is depicted in a variety of shapes, but all of them can be related to the different forms of the plant. In some we see the unique shape of a marijuana leaf. In others the tree appears in a characteristic round shape, or in the conical shape that the plant takes on when it is pruned. There are pictures that show the tree with pendant flowers that are typical of the male of the species. There are pictures of goats consuming the tree and then acting strangely, and there are pictures of hunters trying to keep the goats off the tree. In some scenes, there are images of seated people inhaling through a long straw placed in a bowl at their feet.

To some cultures, including the Celts, the Tree of Life represents the unity of all things. It supports the heavens and connects them to the terrestrial world and, through its roots, to the underworld. Jewish Kabbalists believe the Tree of Life is a diagram illustrating how the universe came into being.

Its branching structure is used to illustrate many cultural concepts including the connection between all forms of creation, the evolutionary divergence of all living creatures, and the migration of ancient populations to new areas.

The seeds of the Tree of Life contain its life essence and represent immortality. The leaves symbolize both physical and spiritual healing and a means to attain long life. For example, in the Hebrew scriptures, stories of Adam, Eve, and a serpent in the Garden of Eden describe the tree's ability to impart immortality. When the Hebrew god Yahweh placed the first man and woman in a garden, he forbade them from eating from the Tree of Knowledge. When a serpent seduces the woman to eat its fruit, and she in turn offers it to the man, God expels them from the garden and thereby from eternal life.

Many Christians believe that the Eucharist, the consecrated bread and wine of their communion ritual, is actually the body and blood of Jesus. The Catholic saints Bonaventure and Albert the Great believed that the Eucharist represents the fruit of the Tree of Life, and that it imparts immortality or the ability to go to "heaven" upon dying.

In Norse mythology, the Tree of Life is also associated with connection to the spirit world, serpents, and sacrifice for knowledge. The Norse Tree connects the nine worlds, and the gods and goddesses live in her branches. The Eagle lives on top of the tree and the World Serpent lives coiled around her roots. The greatest Norse god, Odin, hung himself by his foot in the Tree for nine days and nights so that he would gain knowledge of the mysteries and magic of life.

We also see the symbol of an eagle on top of the Tree of Life and a serpent coiled below it in numerous Asian cosmologies. Asian shamans, like those of Siberia, and others in South America, Africa, and beyond use a Great Tree to ascend to the heavens to communicate with the spirits that live there.

When ancient Sumerians ate fruit from the Tree of Knowledge at Eridu (Eden), the arts of civilization were revealed to them, including writing. They promptly wrote down their religious beliefs and myths and then founded their first city, Urak, which they dedicated to their goddess Innanna.

Ancient Persian and Zoroastrian legends call their Tree of Life *Haoma* and believed it had healing properties when eaten, and its juice was an elixir of immortality. Like modern-day Christians, they believed that a resurrection would occur and those who drank of the life-giving

Haoma juice would obtain perfect welfare, including deathlessness. Magical fish guard this life-giving tree from evil, which continually tries to destroy it, but in this case, evil takes the form of a lizard instead of a serpent.

The Tree of Life exists throughout the ages and in cultures throughout the world, and hemp shares many cosmological attributes with it, including connection, immortality, access to the divine, attainment of knowledge, and physical and spiritual healing. Also, evil forces continuously try to destroy hemp.

But you can't keep a good herb down . . .

CHINA—THE LAND OF *MA* AND MULBERRY (AND EPHEDRA!)

> *First a yin then a yang*
> *No one knows what I do*
> *Jade buds of holy hemp*
> *For the one who lives apart.*
>
> POEM CIRCA 300 BCE
> IN BILL PORTER, *ROAD TO HEAVEN*

Recently discovered evidence indicates that people in China have been getting high for more than 2,500 years. Archaeologists have unearthed a set of ten wooden braziers from eight tombs in what is now China's Xinjiang region, suggesting that they fumigated with pot using bowl-shaped incense burners with small, heated stones.[22] Archeologists debate where the pot came from—was it wild, low-THC hemp? Was it cultivated in the high mountains where it would have developed more THC? Or was it brought in from one of the great trade routes through the area?

Although long known as the Land of Hemp and Mulberry, China is also the home of ephedra, one of the three herbs in the ancient Soma/Haoma recipe. The temples in Bactria-Margiana provided evidence that the Scythians' realm once stretched all the way to northern China. There are fifth-century Chinese documents that refer to an ancient tribe of tall white people with white, yellow, or reddish hair. The ancient Chinese called them the Bai people, and they occupied northwest China in an area now called the Xinjiang, or the Uyghur Autonomous Region, which borders Mongolia, Russia, Kazakhstan, Kyrgyzstan, Tajikistan, Afghanistan, Pakistan, and India. The rest of the world considered these "white Chinese" to be mythical until 1978 when Xinjiang's leading archaeologist, Wang Binghua, made a stunning discovery in caves on the Tien Shan Mountains: mummies with Caucasian features.[23] Since then hundreds more have been found in more than two thousand tombs throughout the region. The caves also hold the shadows of amazing pictographs of ancient shamanic, spirit-altering ceremonies, and the mummies were dressed as Hoama Shamans. They were buried with ephedra and cannabis (some 2,800-year-old buds were still jade green and studded with crystals!) and with stone mortars, beautiful horse chariots, and bronze objects traced back to the Russian steppes. Celtic-style tartan cloth, reminiscent of what we see in traditional Scottish and Irish dress, cowrie shells carried all the way from India, and other Bronze Age artifacts found there indicate a vast, time-worn trading network throughout Europe, the Middle East, and Asia. A closer examination of the Chinese language shows that many Chinese words for things like wheels, spokes, axles, and chariots come from Indo-European languages. Current residents of the region, the Uyghurs, continue to hold the hemp of their Scythian ancestors as a highly valued medicine, and, not coincidentally, they continue to fight for autonomy and freedom from Chinese rule.

Like the Scythian Soma and Haoma cults to the west, Chinese shamans found hemp useful for ridding people of the demons of disease. Hemp offered the power of purity and could conquer evil. These conjurers carved serpents coiled around giant hemp stalks—creating the first known caduceus, a symbol of the physician to this day. Once again, we see the serpent raise her energy to dance with this magical herb!

For thousands of years Chinese shamans pounded on the beds of the afflicted with their magical staff of life and commanded the demons away. As Chinese medicine advanced into the age of herbs and acupuncture around 6000 BCE (before needles, they used sharpened stones and bones), enchanters continued to work with the spirit of hemp and hemp staffs until the Middle Ages.

Paleobotanist Li Hui-lin believes the first cultivation of hemp occurred in a Neolithic village south of Lanchou, where archeologists found a clay pot containing carbonized remains of cultivated hemp buds. According to Li, "Nomad tribes in the north, practitioners of shamanism, apparently used the plant as a drug and carried it west to central and western Asia and India, where it was used primarily as a hallucinogen and not as a textile fiber."[24]

As civilizations in China grew larger, the shamans were pushed into the mountains to live as hermits before eventually fading out altogether. Benjamin Schwartz, author of *The World of Thought in Ancient China*, reiterates a theme we see repeated in many cultures and religions throughout world history: "In the long run, shamanism was not compatible with the emerging religion of the state in China. This religion could not regard with favor a form of individual religious power that by claiming direct access to the divine presumed to bypass the officially sanctioned ritual channels for communicating with divine spirits."[25]

Meanwhile, Daoism began to spread through China as a spiritual philosophy. The Daoist encyclopedia, *Supreme Secret Essentials,* reports that they adapted the religious use of cannabis around 770 BCE. Burning hemp incense was highly valued as a means to achieve immortality and commune with spirits. It still is.

During the Jin Dynasty (265–420 CE) a woman named Wei Huacun founded Shangqing Daoism, which became the dominant school of Daoism throughout the Tang Dynasty (618–907 CE). During her reign, she channeled thirty-one volumes of scriptures from different immortals, or "perfect" men and women, including the Perfect Man of Pristine Emptiness and Perfect Man Jing Lin. These spirits were so impressed with her devotion that they chose to descend and transmit these volumes to her. Scholars agree that the prophetess was most certainly inhaling hemp incense religiously during the process.

Tao Hongjing (456–536 CE), who edited the official Shangqing canon, also compiled the *Mingyi bielu* or "Supplementary Records of Famous Physicians," where we read that cannabis flowers "are very little used in medicine, but the magician-technicians say that if one consumes them with ginseng, it will give one preternatural knowledge of events in the future."[26]

Hemp helped humans develop the arts of spinning and weaving plant fibers into fabric, allowing them to evolve out of animal skins, and people have worn hemp ritually ever since. The oldest preserved piece of hemp fabric was found in an ancient Chinese burial site of the Zhou Dynasty (1046–256 BCE). Hemp garments also played a religious role, according to the ancient Chinese Book of Rites (second century BCE), which stated that mourners must wear hemp clothing out of respect for the dead—a practice continued into modern times. Mulberry, the source of silk, was a fabric only affordable to the very rich. Hemp, once again, clothed the people.

As in all indigenous systems of healing, in China the physical body was married to the spirit and energy of the whole person. The oldest Chinese medical text, the *Pen Ts'ao,* from the first century CE, contains references to hemp, or *ma*, as the "liberator of sin." They knew hemp to possess both yin and yang energy. Illustrating the tolerance factor of THC, the *Pen Ts'ao* also stated that if too many seeds are consumed, they will cause one to see demons, but if used over a long time, they will allow one to communicate with spirits. A later Chinese name for hemp was "delight giver." I still call her that.

There is a lot of linguistic evidence for the ancient Chinese use of hemp as a drug. The Chinese character *ma* is literally a picture of hemp plants drying upside down in a shed. In addition to hemp, it can also mean "numbed," or "tingling." *Ma-tsui* means "hemp-drunk," *ma-mu* (literally "hemp-tree") means "stoned," and *ma-fei-san* ("narcotic bubbling compound") was an anesthetic used for surgery. *Ta ma* is a superior immortality elixir in the Shen Nung pharmacopoeia that caused one to become "a divine transcendent."

In a culture where cannabis has always played a divine role, there is of course a Goddess of Hemp, *Magu*. She is also worshiped in Korea as *Mago* and Japan as *Mako*. Magu is a legendary Daoist immortal associated with health, healing of the universe, and protecting women. Once again, we see cannabis aligned with health and longevity, where the goddess Magu is famous for her Elixir of Life. Often pictured carrying a basket of hemp, she resides on the sacred Mount Tai, a traditional hemp-growing region. Although almost all her shrines and temples were destroyed during the Cultural Revolution in 1966, today one temple to Magu survives on Mount Tai. On the seventh day of the seventh month, when they harvest their hemp, Daoists burn her as incense and hold "séance banquets" at their annual harvest festival to honor Magu.

Legends say that this festival has been held since the beginning of time, "when the world was green. . ."

JAPAN: LAND OF SHAMANS AND SHINTOISM

The history of hemp, or *taima*, in Japan stretches back over ten thousand years and is as rich as its culture. Japan's neolithic period is called the "Jomon Period"—*jomon* means "pattern of ropes."

In Shintoism, Japan's indigenous religion, which is still practiced today, worshipers offer hemp to the gods and use it as a symbol of purity and fertility. Reminiscent of Chinese shamans, Shinto priests perform rites with a short hemp staff, or *gohei,* that has undyed hemp fibers attached to one end representing purity. According to Shinto beliefs, evil and purity cannot exist alongside one another, and so evil spirits are driven out of people by waving the gohei over their heads.

In another old Japanese tradition, they purify their sacred rooms by burning hemp leaves by the entrance. This would invite in the spirits of the departed and encourage people to dance! Buddhists in Japan also burn bundles of taima in their doorways to honor their ancestors and welcome back the spirits of the dead, especially during their annual summer Bon festival. Japanese emperors still wear hemp robes for many ceremonies. Even Sumo wrestlers wear giant hemp rope sashes before a match to purify the ring and exorcize evil spirits. In Shinto shrines and Buddhist temples all over Japan short hempen curtains hang over the doorways to brush evil spirits off the top of the head as one enters.

Hemp was also an integral part of Japanese love and marriage. Strands of hemp are hung on trees as charms to bind lovers and are prominently displayed during wedding ceremonies to symbolize the traditional obedience of Japanese wives to their husbands. Just as hemp is easily dyed different colors, so must wives be "dyed" in any color their husbands chose. The groom's family sent gifts of hemp to the prospective bride's family as a sign that they accepted the bride.

Hemp is offered to the gods in many Japanese traditions. The greatest Shinto goddess, Amaterasu, created the cosmos, all the other gods, and all the hempen clothes they wear. All of Japan's emperors are her descendants and therefore considered divine. Her greatest gift to humans was the art of weaving silk and hemp. She is worshiped with a prayer in which devotees set out taima, salt, and rice at shrines to honor her. She is first among all the gods.

Travelers in Japan made little offerings of taima and rice to protective deities while on journeys. These deities are represented by giant phallus sculptures placed on roadsides and at crossroads around the country to repel malignant spirits.

There is no doubt that the Japanese *kami,* or nature spirits, guided them in becoming some of the world's best farmers, and hemp was one of their favorite crops. Indeed, it was Japanese immigrants who improved farming methods so much in California at the turn of the twentieth century that the state became the breadbasket for the rest of the country. That lasted until the U.S. Farm Security Administration confiscated six thousand farms totaling approximately 200,000 acres during World War II, when all the West Coast's Japanese farmers were forced into internment camps. Japanese hemp strains being grown at that time outperformed those in Europe and China for height, stem strength, length of internodes, and quality and quantity of fiber.[27]

They also produced more THC, according to a United Nations Office on Drugs and Crime report in 1973, which found THC levels of 3.9 percent as opposed to American varieties that clocked in at 1.5 percent at that time.

In ancient Japan, women perfected hemp-processing techniques. They developed a three-step water retting method, an alkaline bleaching method, and wove cloth as fine as silk. Whereas the upper class monopolized sake (a Japanese rice wine), cannabis, once again, was the drug of choice for the commoners.

Hemp was completely intertwined with Japanese culture, philosophy, and religion until the U.S. occupation forces outlawed it after WWII. This was a precursor to the government outlawing marijuana in the United States to (once again) subjugate a class of people. According to Junichi Takayasu, a Japanese hemp rights advocate and considered one of Japan's leading experts on cannabis,

> In a mere half century, MacArthur, with the Hemp Control Act, managed to totally wipe away even the memories of hemp culture, which had endured for several thousand years . . . In the same way that U.S. authorities discouraged kendo and judo, the 1948 Cannabis Control Act was a way to undermine militarism in Japan . . . The wartime cannabis industry had been so dominated by the military that the Cannabis Control Act was designed to strip away its power. The struggle to liberate and revive hemp is therefore a struggle to renew Japanese culture and liberate the country from the occupation policies and colonial subjugation of the United States. Speaking spiritually, I believe this struggle is every bit as important as the movement in Okinawa today for the removal of the American bases. We are talking about physical and spiritual independence.[28]

Today, most Japanese believe that cannabis is a narcotic and do not even realize that it is the same plant as hemp. But it's hard to keep a good herb down . . .

THE HEBREWS: TRADERS AND TRAVELERS

Most Westerners of any religion are culturally aware of the most famous myths and characters in the Bible. But few are aware that the biblical priests and prophets all used cannabis. Cannabis has been found at 2,800-year-old Jewish temple sites.[29] Even Jesus partook of this magical Tree of Life. There are references and recipes for cannabis throughout the Bible, and both the Hebrew scriptures and the Christian scriptures teach us how to use cannabis to commune with their gods.

The Hebrew scriptures mention cannabis, which the ancient Hebrews called *kaneh-bosm*, or sometimes just *kaneh,* five times: in Exodus, the Song of Songs, Isaiah, Jeremiah, and Ezekiel. It is called both spirit-altering incense and healing anointing oils. The ancient Jewish tribes were very active in the cannabis incense trades occurring throughout the region, along with, no surprise, the Scythians. "Danites and Greeks from Uzal bought your merchandise; They exchanged wrought iron, cassia and kaneh for your Wares."[30]

The god of the Israelites loved this magical incense so much that he demanded its presence at all times and became quite grumpy when it was not provided. See, for example, Exodus 30:8–10: "And Aaron shall burn incense every morning: When he dresseth the lamps, he shall burn incense upon it. And when Aaron lighteth the lamps at eve, he shall burn incense upon it, a perpetual incense before the Lord throughout your generations." Or another example in Isaiah 43:23–24: "You have not brought any Kaneh for me, or lavished on me the fat of your sacrifices. But you have burned me with your sins and wearied me with your offenses."

An etymologist named Sula Benet established the ancient Hebrews' use of cannabis in 1936. She showed that the Semitic word *kaneh-bosm* is the origin of the word *cannabis.* Why have you never heard of this? Because kaneh-bosm had been mistranslated as "calamus" in the oldest Greek translation of the Hebrew scriptures in the third century BCE. The error was repeated in the many translations that followed—sometimes again mistranslated to "fragrant cane" or simply "reed." Imagine what Jewish and Christian society might be today without that blunder![31]

In the Exodus story in the Torah, when Moses initially encountered an angel from his god, the angel spoke from within a burning bush and proceeded to tell Moses to lead his people to freedom! Once again, cannabis and ideas of liberation could be linked.

The next references to kaneh involve that same shaman-prophet, Moses, and a magical anointing oil. In Exodus 30:22–30 (King James version), Moses receives instructions to make a sacred anointing oil. Although the formula is suspiciously like oils used in Egypt at that time, in the Torah, the recipe is given to Moses by God himself! "Moreover the Lord spake unto Moses, saying, take thou also unto thee principal spices, of pure myrrh five hundred shekels, and of sweet cinnamon half so much, even two hundred and fifty shekels, and of sweet calamus [kaneh-bosum] two hundred and fifty shekels, and of cassia five hundred shekels, after the shekel of the sanctuary, and of oil olive an hin: And thou shalt make it an oil of holy ointment, an ointment compound after the art of the apothecary: it shall be an holy anointing oil. . . And thou shalt anoint Aaron and his sons, and consecrate them, that they may minister unto me in the priest's offices."

Translated into modern-day measurements, Moses was extracting about *nine pounds* of kaneh into one hin of olive oil. That's a mere 6.5 liters (less than 2 gallons) of olive oil—medicine strong enough to get an ox high!

Yahweh goes on to express an extreme affection, or shall we say need, for this spirit-altering drug. He instructs his prophet to use it to anoint the tabernacle. This means Moses was actually rubbing down the walls of a tent with very psychoactive oil. He was also to anoint not only all the holy vessels, but himself as well. This all occurred in the desert heat, where Moses was bound to absorb THC through his sweat-opened pores. His god also told him to fumigate the tabernacle, equivalent to hotboxing the tent, which would indicate that every time this Levite priest heard his god speak, he was likely thoroughly stoned.

Contributing to a worldwide theme, the use of this intoxicating oil was restricted to the priesthood, and later for the initiation of the patriarchal royalty of the Jewish kingdoms, in order that they and no others might "receive the revelations of the Lord." The royals were referred to as Messiah-Kings. The Hebrew word *Messiah* (like the Greek word *Christ*) means "one who has been anointed."

As in the story of Soma, after the fall of the kingdoms of Israel between 700 and 400 BCE, the sacred and powerful kaneh-bosm anointing oil was prohibited and the use of cannabis in worship fell from grace. Patriarchy and its authoritarian monotheism were on the rise and forcibly stamping out all matriarchal goddess religions and polytheism—including the cult of Asherah.

Ashera, the wife/consort of Yahweh, was also worshiped with hemp incense and oils. And Jeremiah, for one, made note of the consequences of ignoring her (Jeremiah 44:18): "But ever since we stopped burning incense to the Queen of Heaven and pouring out drink offerings to her, we have had nothing and have been perishing by sword and famine."

There is little to no reference to kaneh-bosm in the rest of the Old Testament, and after the reference in Jeremiah, Ashera is referred to as the Tree of Life, the Tree of Knowledge, or a grove of trees. Thus, due to mistaken translations in the English King James Bible, one of the most printed books in the world, English language readers were never exposed to the existence of cannabis as a sacrament, or the great goddess Asherah.

But as is probably clear by now, you can't keep a good herb down!

CHRISTIANITY: JESUS THE ANOINTED ONE

Cannabis rose again, and it was Jesus himself who resurrected the herb this time, and then, unlike his predecessors, he gave it to the people!

A truly surprising number of stories featuring holy kaneh-bosm are to be found in both the Christian scriptures and the Gnostic texts. The Gnostic texts are recently discovered ancient gospels written by a sect of Christians in the second and third centuries after Jesus lived. They were lost from the third century until 1945 when they were found in a desert cave in Egypt by two brothers who were digging there for fertilizer. They were probably purposefully hidden by the Gnostic Christians because the Orthodox Christians were burning everything that contradicted their "official" version of Jesus's teachings, and these writings include many gospels about Jesus. According to cannabis historian Chris Bennett: "There is no reason to consider these ancient Gnostic documents as less accurate portrayals of the life and teachings of Jesus than the New Testament. The rediscovery of the texts marks the resurrection of Jesus as an ecstatic rebel sage who preached enlightenment through rituals involving magical plants."[32]

Contrary to the accounts of Matthew and Luke, written twelve generations after Jesus's death, in the Gnostic view Jesus did not become the "Messiah" until John the Baptist initiated him. Gnostic texts reveal that John performed his baptisms not only with water but in conjunction with a kaneh-bosm anointing oil ritual. It was this act that made Jesus a *Christ,* or "anointed one."

Isaiah 61:1–2 says that upon being anointed, Jesus exclaimed: "The Spirit of Yahweh god is upon me, because Yahweh has anointed me to bring good tidings to the afflicted; He has sent me to bind up the brokenhearted, to proclaim liberty to the captives and to open the prison of those who are bound."

This enlightened wandering ascetic prophet began preaching freedom and happiness the minute he experienced cannabis for the first time! Unlike Moses and Soma, he did not keep this newfound power to himself but spread it throughout his world as quickly as possible. First, he anointed his disciples then sent them out to anoint the people (Mark 6:13): "And they cast out many devils, and anointed with oil many that were sick, and healed them."

This created an ever-increasing group of enlightened ones, soon to be called "Christians," the plural form of the word *christ.* Jesus preached that one did not need a priest or rabbi to reach God but would know God via the anointing ritual and remain forevermore endowed with all knowledge (John 2:27): "But the anointing which ye have received of him abideth in you, and ye need not that any man teach you: but as the same anointing teacheth you of all things, and is truth, and is no lie."

Here we have both another reference to cannabis bringing knowledge and wisdom to the people and perhaps a new perspective on the many stories of Jesus and his disciples performing miracles and healing people. With the laying on of hands coated with cannabis-infused oil, Jesus is reported to have healed wounds and straightened crooked limbs, cured leprosy, and caused the blind to see. There is even a Bible story of Jesus healing chronic menstrual problems! Injuries, arthritis, skin diseases, glaucoma, painful periods—was it Jesus or marijuana that performed these miracles?

And like the ancient Soma, Christian cannabis also held the power to relieve sin (James 5:13–15): "Is anyone among you sick? Let them call the elders of the church to pray over them and anoint them with oil in the name of the Lord. And the prayer offered in faith will make the sick person well; The Lord will raise them up. If they have sinned, they will be forgiven."

INDIA: LAND OF BHANG, BUDDHA, SIKHS, AND SHIVA

When priests and magi restricted the ritual use of cannabis to the powerful, its use seemed to die out when religious values changed. However, the worship of hemp has never actually died but merely headed underground to morph and resurface in a different form. In the case of the death of Soma, or Indra's food, sacred cannabis sprang forth again later in the form of the god Shiva.

Shiva is the Hindu god of cannabis, or *bhang*. Artifacts and archaic clay figurines of Shiva illustrate that people worshiped her/him six thousand years before Jesus was born, and they continue to do so today. Like Soma, the word *Bhang* refers to the hemp plant, the sacred tea made from it, and to Lord Shiva her/himself. It is said that "He who drinks Bhang drinks Shiva."

So, Bhang is not just a sacred bridge *to the divine*, it *is the divine!* That makes cannabis the oldest continually worshiped divine being on Earth!

As She Makes Bhang . . .

She takes a handful of the fresh, green herb
and crushes it in her fist
as she inhales the uplifting, heady aroma.
Into the mortar they go
with a splash of fresh milk.
She sprinkles in poppy seeds
and a few slices of ginger.
She begins to pray for her family
as she pounds the herbs using her favorite old pestle
in a quiet rhythm
entrained with her heartbeat.
She squeezes the golden green liquid from the mash,
adds more milk,
and returns to her rhythmic pressing.
In another mortar she begins to pound black pepper,
turning her head away
to avoid the sharp aroma.
She adds some sweet-smelling caraway seeds
and a few spicy cloves
and begins to pound in a more upbeat tempo.
In go pungent cardamom pods,
along with some cinnamon chips
and dried cucumber seeds.
Nutmeg!
She brings a carefully wrapped paper pouch
from her apron
and unties the pretty ribbon
to reveal three shiny nuts
the spice seller got from the harbor just yesterday.
She grates one and scatters a pinch into the mortar.
Again, a splash of milk.
She continues to pound, splash, and press—

slowly turning the slurry into tea.
Then everything is warmed
in her great-grandmother's teapot—
it is far too chilly a night to serve cold bhang!
She changes hands while stirring the tea,
thereby changing the direction
of the gentle vortex inside.
With a ladle she lifts some to her lips for a test.
Not satisfied,
she lifts the conical top
from a brightly colorful ceramic urn
and brings out three more bundles
of the magic green leaves.
An extra bunch for Uncle's aching knees,
a bunch for Mother and Father who are fighting again.
And for her?
A bunch for her to let her mind float
toward holy things on this holy day . . .
She adds sugar to bring sweetness,
and as her loved ones gather to celebrate Shiva's Day,
she serves them her prayer
in fine china cups
with pink rose petals floating on top
for love.

The Creation of Bhang—The Churning of the Ocean of Milk

In this story, Indra, King of the Gods, was riding his mighty elephant in a long, colorful procession through the streets. The god Shiva was in the watching crowd and threw an offering up to Indra—a beautiful, glowing garland of sacred marigolds that he had threaded himself. Indra caught the golden gift and, without a second glance, tossed it to his mighty ride. When the elephant promptly stomped on it, the trouble really began.

Shiva in his rage cursed the King of the Gods, and, suddenly, all the gods became weak. With their power diminished, the demons seized the advantage and challenged the deities. A great war broke out, lasting twelve long years. Well, twelve long god-years, but 144 human-years.

At this point the weary gods traveled to the primordial ocean, the Sea of Milk, to pray to Vishnu, the Tamer of Demons. Vishnu led them in preparing *amrita*, the "nectar of immortality." He told the gods to use a sacred mountain, Mandara, as a giant churning stick, and Vasuki, the king of the serpents, as a rope so that they could churn the sea to make amrita. However, the mountain was so magnificent that they could not turn the churning stick by themselves—they had to have the demons' help! But how would they keep the demons from stealing the amrita, that sweet nectar of immortality?

Vishnu had a plan. With the gods pulling the tail of the mighty snake wrapped around the sacred mountain, and the demons pulling his head, slowly the mountain began to stir the Ocean of Milk. Under Vishnu's direction, the gods tossed "potent herbs" into the sea, and her treasures began to rise to the surface. The first blessing to rise was Surabhi, the wish-bestowing cow, followed by the Goddess of Wine, the Tree of Paradise, and then the moon, which Shiva placed upon his brow. A great poison also came forth, threatening the world, which Shiva drank down—thereby saving the world, although it turned him blue.

Then sprang forth the most precious treasure: Dhanvantari, the shaman of the gods was born, holding a milk-white chalice, or *khumba*, of amrita, the Dew of Life.

Of course, the demons immediately stole it. The whole world was in danger of the demons becoming immortal! But Vishnu was prepared, for he knew demons well, and he sent a bird to steal back the khumba of amrita. The gods drank the amrita and became reinvigorated. Using their renewed strength, they drove the demons to hell.

And while the bird was in flight with that khumba, everywhere drops of the precious amrita spilled to the ground and a beautiful bhang plant sprang forth! For this reason, bhang is called *viyasha*, or "victorious," and to this day, whenever I see a bhang plant, I know that some dew of life has fallen there from the heavens.

Hindu holy people, called *sadhus,* and Shiva worshipers from all over the world still celebrate the creation of bhang at a festival named for that sacred chalice—Kumbha Mela. Every three years at one of four sacred spots where amrita spilled and bhang sprang up, millions gather to celebrate at the largest religious gathering in the world. Every 144 years, there is a Great Kumbha Mela festival. The last one was in 2001, and 60 million souls attended—the largest gathering of humans ever recorded, all brought together by cannabis.

Ganga, Shiva, and Ganja

There is an area of the Himalayas that is believed to be Shiva reclining. His long locks of hair flow across India forming her great rivers. When the great Goddess Ganga wished to come to Earth from the heavens, Shiva worried that she would flood the world, so he caught her in his long wild locks as she fell to the ground and calmed her to a manageable flow. She became the Ganges River, the most sacred river in India, and perhaps the world. The flow of that river represents both the Goddess Ganga and bhang, the nectar of immortality. The Himalayas that are the river's source grow huge amounts of hemp, called ganja. The Ganges River also flows through Bangladesh, an ancient city named for the god-plant Bhang.

Shiva drank bhang when it was created during the churning of the Ocean of Milk and has been perpetually intoxicated ever since. At one time, this upset his wife, Parvathi, and they fought. Shiva left and went into the fields to be by himself. He took shelter from the blazing sun under a hemp plant and crushed and ate some of the leaves. The bhang refreshed him so completely he took it as his favorite food and became the "Lord of Bhang." He shared it with his wife, and they then made bhang together.

As many a modern-day cultivator can tell you, growing pot is a spiritual experience. What they may not realize is that Shiva taught us this six thousand years ago! When Shiva instructed Parvathi to grow bhang, he insisted on the following ritual:

In sowing hemp seed, you should keep repeating the spell "Bhangi," "Bhangi," . . . the sound of that guardian name may scare the evil influences. Again, when the seedlings are planted the same holy name must be repeated, and also at the watering which, for the space of a year, the young plants must daily receive. When the flowers appear the flowers and leaves should be stripped from the plant and kept for a day in warm water. The next day, with one hundred repetitions of the holy name Bhangi, the leaves and flowers should be washed in a river and dried in an open shed. When they are dry some of the leaves should be burnt with due repeating of the holy name as a charm. Then, bearing in mind Vagdevata, the goddess of speech, and offering a prayer, the dried leaves should be laid in a pure and sanctified place. Bhang so prepared, especially if prayers are said over it, will gratify the wishes and desires of its owner.[33]

As an act of worship, many Hindus pour bhang over a sculpted *linga* (lingam) of Shiva. The bhang is captured in the *yoni* receptacle on which it sits. The linga is symbolic of the penis and the generative power of Lord Shiva. The yoni represents the receptive vagina, and together they signify the union of male and female powers in nature. You will find linga/yoni altars at temples and in public places throughout India.

Sadhus

India has large populations of sadhus, holy people and wandering ascetics who worship Shiva. *Sadhu* is a Sanskrit term that means "to practice something with complete dedication and a single pointed focus to the exclusion of all else." Sadhus renounce family and all other ties to place, community, and caste to become completely free to pursue a spiritual quest. Like Shiva, they love to smoke pot out of clay *chillums,* or pipes, as a part of their devotional practice. They cover themselves with dust and ashes as a reminder of ever-present death, and they wear long, unkempt dreadlocks, like their god.

The Indians venerate sadhus. To be in the presence of a holy one is to be in the presence of celestial radiance. To even *see* one is considered a sacred sign. They earn their rice by begging, and it is a divine blessing for people to fill their bowls. In complete contradiction to Western societies' view of sadhus as dirty, long-haired, pot-smoking beggars, Indians believe that "the mere sight of bhang cleanses from as much sin as a thousand horse-sacrifices or a thousand pilgrimages. He who scandalizes the user of bhang shall suffer the torments of hell so long as the sun endures."[34]

The holy ones extoll and glorify Bhang because she facilitates a higher vision of reality and easy communication with the divine. Like Soma, Bhang is "a sure way of attaining divine wisdom." Bhang is believed to cleanse the body of sin. Like the Christian communion ritual where to consume bread is to consume the body of Jesus, the devotee who partakes of bhang partakes of the god Shiva. "This bhang Shiva made from his own body..." is how the India Hemp Drugs Commission reported it in the early 1890s. Today the worship of Shiva is one of the three most influential denominations in contemporary Hinduism. In addition to Bhang, Shiva is also the Lord of Hashish, or *charas*. He is often invoked before taking the first puff of ganja from a chillum.

The Sikhs

The founder of the Indian Sikh religion was a great warrior guru called Singh. One day, when he was leading his troops in a critical skirmish, his soldiers suddenly panicked at the sight of an enemy's elephant bearing down on them with a sword in its trunk! The giant beast was slashing its way through the men like butter, and they were diving away from it in every direction, on the verge of breaking rank. Singh feared a disastrous rout. He needed a man willing to risk certain death to slay the maniacal elephant. So, he created one. Grabbing the man closest to him, he poured some bhang and a little opium down his throat and set him to the task. Fortified by the drug, the loyal soldier rushed into the thick of battle and charged the elephant. Deftly evading its slashing blows, he managed to slip under the elephant and with all his strength plunge his weapon into its unprotected belly. When Singh's men saw the elephant lying dead, they rallied and overpowered the enemy. From that time forth, the Sikhs commemorate the anniversary of that great battle by drinking bhang.

Tantra

Tantra, which emerged as a philosophy in India in the seventh century, weaves together ancient Shiva-worshiping Hinduism and Tibetan Buddhism. Worshipers seek altered states of consciousness through cannabis, yoga, and sex. They seek to commune with their own divine nature to work toward attaining *nirvana*, the ultimate Buddhist goal. Cannabis, of course, plays a preeminent part in Tantra by heightening awareness, enhancing sex, and facilitating a deeper yoga and meditation practice. One of the tantric texts, Yoga Sutra 4.1, describes the process: "The subtler attainments come with birth or are attained through herbs, mantra, austerities or concentration."

Tantric Buddhists believe that Buddha subsisted for six years on nothing but hemp seeds. In another important tantric text, the *Mahanirvana Tantra*, Shiva explains his love of bhang to his female side, Shakti: "For thy pleasure, O Beloved! I shall speak of that which is dearer to me than even life itself. To all sufferings it brings relief. It wards off all dangers. It gives Thee pleasure, and it is the way by which Thou art most swiftly obtained. For men rendered wretched by the taint of the Kali Age, short-lived and unfit for strenuous effort, this is the greatest wealth."[35]

The British Meet Bhang

While ruling India, the British invented the gin and tonic—I will be forever grateful!—and they also sponsored what is still the most extensive, comprehensive, and qualitative research ever done on the influence of cannabis on a society. Looking to make bhang illegal, they set up a commission to study its effects, and the result was *The India Hemp Drug Commission Report of 1894*. The Commission interviewed nearly two thousand informants across India and Burma, including European medical officers, native healers, cultivators, traders, and others. The British colonial bureaucrats produced a lucid and timeless report on the effects of cannabis on the mind, body, and morality of the people of India.

Many decades later, an American doctor named Tod Hiro Mikuriya came across the report while he was studying cannabis and mentioned it in his book *Marijuana Medical Papers 1839–1972*, characterizing it as "comprising some seven volumes and 3,281 pages . . . by far the most complete and systematic study of marijuana undertaken to date."[36]

The following quotations from the report, in which cannabis is referred to as bhang, indicate its tenor and scope:

> The quickening spirit of bhang is the spirit of freedom and knowledge. In the ecstasy of bhang the spark of the Eternal in man turns into light the murkiness of matter.

> Not a single one has ever observed the use giving rise to mental aberration, the use of hemp drugs is practically attended by no evil results at all. . . . no injurious effects on the mind. . . . no moral injury whatever.

> To the Hindu the hemp plant is holy. . . A guardian . . . the bhang leaf is the home of Shiva.

> No god or man is as good as the religious drinker of bhang.

> Sanctified bhang taken at day break or noon destroys disease.

> That a day may be fortunate the careful man should on waking look into liquid bhang . . . So any nightmares or evil spirits that may have entered into him during the ghost-haunted hours of night will flee from him at the sight of the bhang and free him from their blinding influences during the day.

> To meet someone carrying bhang is a sure omen of success. To see in a dream the leaves, plant, or water of bhang is lucky; it brings the goddess of wealth into the dreamer's power.

> Pardeshi or North Indian Hindus of Bombay . . . who fails to give his visitor bhang is despised by his caste as mean and miserly.

Bhang the cooler is a febrifuge . . . indirectly or spiritually by soothing the angry influences to whom the heats of fever are due.

Soothes the over-wakeful to sleep, gives beauty, and secures length of days, makes the tongue of the lisper plain, freshens the intellect, and gives alertness to the body and gaiety to the mind.

Bhang, deepens thought, and braces judgment.

Raising man out of himself and above mean individual worries, makes him one with the divine force of nature.

Bhang is the spirit of freedom and knowledge.

Clearer of ignorance, the giver of knowledge. No gem or jewel can touch in value bhang.

Much of the holiness of bhang is due to its virtue of clearing the head and stimulating the brain to thought.

He who drinks bhang drinks Shiva. The soul in whom the spirit of bhang finds a home glides into the ocean of Being freed from the weary round of matter-blinded self.

Bhang is the Joy-giver, the Sky-flier, the Heavenly-guide, the Poor Man's Heaven, the Soother of Grief.

A plant that became holy from its guardian and healing qualities.

According to one account, when nectar was produced from the churning of the ocean, something was wanted to purify the nectar. The deity supplied the want of a nectar-cleanser by creating bhang. This bhang Shiva made from his own body.

He who uses no bhang shall lose his happiness in this life and in the life to come. In the end he shall be cast into hell. The mere sight of bhang cleanses from as much sin as a thousand horse-sacrifices or a thousand pilgrimages. He who scandalizes the user of bhang shall suffer the torments of hell so long as the sun endures.

No good thing can come to the man who treads under-foot the holy bhang leaf.

Besides over the demon of Madness, bhang is Vijaya, or victorious, over the demons of hunger and thirst. The supporting power of bhang has brought many a Hindu family safe through the miseries of famine.

To forbid or even seriously to restrict the use of so holy and gracious an herb as the hemp would cause widespread suffering and annoyance and to the large bands of worshiped ascetics deep-seated anger. It would rob the people of a solace in discomfort, of a cure in sickness, of a guardian whose gracious protection saves them from the attacks of evil influences, and whose mighty power makes the devotee of the Victorious, overcoming the demons of hunger and thirst, of panic fear, of the glamour of Maya or matter, and of madness, able in rest to brood on the Eternal, till the Eternal, possessing him body and soul, frees him from the haunting of self and receives him into the ocean of Being.

Derived from the ancient god Soma, Bhang and her representative, Lord Shiva, have been worshiped in India for over six thousand years, since she was first brought across the mountains from Persia. Oh, and the British never did outlaw bhang!

PERSIA: LAND OF THE SUFIS

In a monastery that he built deep in the mighty mountains of Persia, there lived a Muslim Sufi called Haydar. An ascetic with a disciplined inner focus, for ten years he rarely left the sanctuary until, one year, he experienced a desperate depression coupled with a longing that was driving him down and keeping him there. Fleeing his inner turmoil, he left the stone temple and wandered off into the surrounding fields to be alone.

After years of deep prayer and inner reflection, he lifted his eyes to the world around—the bright cloudless sky and broad meadows oppressed into stillness by the midday heat. Not a breeze stirred, nor a rodent scratched in the dirt. Insects sang out their songs, but the birds were silent. All was motionless, except for one plant.

One giant, emerald-green plant joyfully dancing under the influence of the midday sun! Surely, this was a sign from Allah! Drawn to it, Haydar fell to his knees in wonder. He picked some leaves, crushed them, and inhaled. What aroma! It cleared his senses and lifted his heart. Chewing them brought on a euphoria he had never experienced before.

Upon his return to the monastery, his disciples immediately noticed the change in his demeanor. Astounded, they began celebrating even as they crowded around him begging for his insight. He made them swear an oath of secrecy not to reveal what he was about to share. "God almighty has granted you as a special favour, an awareness of the virtues of this leaf, so that your use of it will dissipate the cares that obscure your souls and free your spirits from everything that might hamper them, keep carefully, then the deposit he has confided in you."[37]

After ten more years of monastic teaching and sharing the secret of happiness with all Sufis, Haydar passed on. He requested that seeds of his holy plant be sown around his tomb so that even in death he might enjoy the shade of its leaves and scent of its flowers. From there, the Sufis' discovery of cannabis migrated into Iraq, Syria, and Egypt, where it became known as Haydar's Lady and the Wine of Haydar.

ISLAM: ON THE FRINGE

"Hemp . . . as an intoxicant . . . was passed on via Persians, to the Arabs," according to historian Andrew Sherratt.[38] Fringe Islamic sects like the Sufis and the Ismailis have carried on the ancient traditional sacramental use of bhang. As with the Tantra-practicing yogis, Islamic Sufis attain spiritual insights by creating ecstatic states. They believe that divine truth and communion with Allah cannot be imparted to others, rather it must be experienced directly. They worship with cannabis to stimulate mystical consciousness and gain otherwise unattainable insights into themselves. With hashish they see new and different meanings in what appear to be otherwise trivial experiences. They see beautiful colors and designs in what seems commonplace to others. Bhang enhances their pleasure in music and relieves their worries. Simply put, she brings them happiness.

An eighth-century Islamic sect called the Ismailians left us this line of poetry: "We've quaffed the emerald cup, the mystery we know, / Who'd dream so weak a plant such mighty power could show!"[39]

Other medieval Islamic names for cannabis give us an inkling of how her devotees felt about her:

the one that cheers	shrub of understanding
shrub of emotion	girlfriend
peace of mind	the one that connects the heart
the one that facilitates digestion	branches of bliss
the pleasing one	thought morsel
provisions	medicine
the one that lightens the load	sugary
holy Jerusalem	the pretty one
medicinal powder	theriac (heal-all)
peacocks' tail	consolation
the one that causes good appetite	the one that softens the
the one that brings the party	temperaments
together	the little agent
amber scented	from Zion
little morsel	emerald mine[40]

The Arabs gave her the name *kif,* a word for a state of deep mental and spiritual awareness or dreamy tranquility. It comes from the Arabic word *kayf,* which means "pleasure."

Some ancient Muslim cultures also connected Ashera and the Tree of Life.

In light of Ashera's recognition as a symbol of the sacred tree and her cult's use of cannabis (Emboden 1972), it is of interest to note that in medieval times, certain Moslem groups, referred to cannabis by the name *ashirah,* seen by them as an endearing term for their hempen *girlfriend* (Rosenthal 1971), a tradition likely carried on from the earlier association of the ancient goddess and the Tree of Life, in the form of cannabis hemp.[41]

There are stories of the great Islamic prophet Muhammad using bhang. In one story, he used his turban to filter the green tea, which turned his turban green. His hereditary clan, the Bini Hashim, still wear green turbans today.

Many other Sufis, faqirs, mendicants, and mystics who follow the tenants of Islam love hashish and utilize it in their spiritual practices. In their poetry, Bektashi dervishes frequently describe hashish and opium as paths to paradise and the divine.[42] The Islamic world even has a Patron Saint of Cannabis named Khizr, the Green One.

Invaders and colonial influences in the nineteenth century led to a considerable decline in the social approval of ganja-based religions, and although they still play an important part in the Islamic community, they are often forced to the edges of society, and some Muslims hold them in disdain. That said, it's still hard to keep a good herb down!

AFRICA: LAND OF DAGGA

Somewhere around the first millennium before the Common Era, Cannabis got restless. Having fully explored Asia and the Middle East on the backs of Scythian horses, she was looking for a new scene. So, she decided to hitch a ride with some Arab sailors and go explore Africa. What fun it was—sailing across the Arabian Sea! These merchant marines loved her because she quelled their seasick stomachs and gave them better night vision for following the stars. On one of those boat rides she befriended Coffee, and they went on to tour North Africa together. They were seen at all the cafes and kiosks, where the Muslims eschewed beer, wine, and the modern distilled alcohol. She played with all the great musicians, artists, and poets. In the women's chambers and harems, she eased the pain of menstruation and childbirth and led them in prayer. Alongside her friend Coffee she inspired great conversations and debates—and often on those occasions, discussion turned to the quest for freedom.

It was in sub-Saharan Africa, around 600 BCE, that she inspired the invention of the pipe. Not content to sip her as tea, or to blindly try to inhale her incense from a smoky tent, the Africans found a way to bring her pure essence directly into their lungs. With the hollow straws of bones and reeds, and bowls of nuts and clay, they fashioned two kinds of pipes: the water pipe and the dry pipe. These new smoking methods significantly changed her influence, making it stronger and faster acting.

The Portuguese, colonizers of today's Angola and Mozambique, use the word *cachimbo* for pipe. They coined the term in the 1500s, when they invaded dagga-loving regions around the Great Zambezi River. Several local languages from there share terms for dry pipes like the Chichewa *kachimbo* or Tonga *katsimbu*. The loanword *cachimbo* then found its way into Spanish and French.

When Cannabis reached the year-round all-day sun of the equator, she really took off. No longer held back by the Eurasian temperate climates and short growing seasons, now she was able to reach her full potential, reaching heights of ten or twelve feet. She narrowed her leaves so as not to get burnt and began producing more THC.

And she kept traveling spreading herself and her magic all over Africa, a continent bigger than Asia, Europe, Australia, and the Americas combined. She traveled by foot, by camel, by river boat, and with the slave trade, easing the slaves' sorrow as they plodded across that vast continent. The slaves carried her all the way to Western Africa—where she again reached the sea. From the Wolof tribe of Senegal, south to the BaKongo people of Angola, everywhere she arrived she was instantly loved and rapidly adopted into the tribe. The Ambundu of the Congo, a matriarchal tribe, gave her the name *mariamba,* which the Portuguese invaders pronounced *marihuana.*

She headed south with the Bantu tribes as they migrated to where the Atlantic and the Indian Oceans meet. She became a beloved of the hunter-gatherer tribes. The Khoikhoi and San people loved her because she gave them the patience to be good predators and helped them commune with the spirits of nature. They named her Dagga—a moniker she proudly carries today in Southern Africa.

Much later, in the mid-nineteenth century, Cannabis inspired a whole new religion among a tribe who called themselves the *Bena Riamba*, or the Sons of Marihuana. Like the marijuana-inspired hippies a hundred years later, the youth of the tribe wanted to cease a long tribal history of wars and feuds. They found that Riamba promoted peace and friendship among old enemies, and it inspired them to overthrow their elder leaders and ban weapons in their villages. They greeted each other with the word *moyo*, which meant "life" or "health," and invited Mariamba into their rituals, gatherings, and ceremonies, including the celebration of new alliances. The Bena Riamba were an example of the social-cultural transformations that called for peace and unity that swept through Central Africa at the time. Unfortunately, when the Belgians conquered the area and suppressed the movement, the area once again dissolved into political and ethnic conflict.[43]

A Timeless Story

The industry had been thriving for years and the farmers and their families were reaping considerable profits from the green herb that grew like a weed. The merchants were swelling the villages with new shops and buildings, and all were flourishing from this plant that gave freely of its medicine and mysticism alike.

But the ancient Egyptian government still did not like this plant that gave people visions of freedom and oneness, and they began to crack down once again. Growers and merchants could afford to bribe the officials, and so for a while it was back to business as usual.

Until 1378 CE, that is, when an order came down to destroy the hemp fields once and for all. But this time, the farmers united and chose to resist. The governor sent troops into the fields intent on total decimation.

Determined to preserve their livelihoods, the farmers secured their fields, and the troops were forced to back off and eventually decided to place the whole area under siege and hopefully starve the growers into submission.

The people held out for several months, but the soldiers finally broke through the village defenses and there was no alternative but to capitulate. The valley was placed under martial law. They torched the fields, placed many towns under strict surveillance, and razed others to the ground. They shuttered local cannabis cafes and hashish kiosks. Proprietors of these businesses were hunted down and killed. Patrons of these shops and all known hashish users were assembled in the town squares, and in full view of all the townspeople, soldiers wrenched out their teeth.

However, by 1393 CE, the hashish business would once again come back and thrive. Because you can't keep a good herb down! It is a good and mighty thing that you can't keep a good herb down . . .

JAMAICA: LAND OF GANJA AND THE RASTAFARIANS

Once upon a time, the Queen of Sheba, great-granddaughter of Noah, left her home in present day Ethiopia to visit the Holy Land of Jerusalem, where she met King Solomon, who impressed her so much that she adopted his Jewish religion and carried it back to Africa. But that was not all that she took home with her—she was also carrying King Solomon's child, and with his birth came the birth of a new religion—Falasha—the religion of black Jews.

Menelik I was the founder of the House of Solomon, a dynasty that ruled Ethiopia off and on until 1974. The last emperor of the dynasty, Ras Tafari, was crowned Haile Selassie I in 1930. He was a direct descendant of King Solomon and the 225th king in that line.

His followers also refer to him as "the Lion of Judah" and "King of Kings, Lord of Lords." Some believe that he was the second coming of Jesus the Messiah.

Meanwhile, in the West Indies, a new cannabis religion was born on the island of Jamaica. From India, cannabis, known as *ganja*, caught a ride to Jamaica with East Indian indentured slaves in the late 1800s. The herbalists quickly adopted her and served her as tea, and people also blended her with tobacco from the new world and smoked her. By 1930 she had infused herself into the culture and inspired yet another new religion, Rastafarianism, named for the newly crowned emperor of Ethiopia.

With a mix of Judeo-Christian beliefs, Rastafarians follow their own unique version of the Bible because they believe that the white power structure (called Babylon) distorted the standard Bible in order to oppress Africans. They believe that King Solomon, and therefore the Israelites, were black and that as descendants of a black Solomon and a black Queen of Sheba they are one of the lost tribes of Israel. They also believe that Ras Tafari was the born-again Messiah that one of their leaders, Marcus Garvey, had predicted. It is fascinating to note that even though Emperor Selassie refused the claim and died in 1974 at the hands of a military coup, many Rastafarians still believe that he is the savior. Like common views about Jesus, they believe his death was a hoax.

Rastafarians also believe that ganja is a holy herb and the Tree of Life. They note that she is sanctioned many times in the Bible. For example, in Revelation (22:2): "In the midst of the street, and on either side of the river, was there the tree of life, which bore twelve manner of fruits, and yielded her fruit every month: and the leaves of the tree were for the healing of the nations." And again in Psalms (104:14): "He causeth the grass to grow for the cattle, and herb for the service of man that he may bring forth food out of the earth."

Rastafarians believe that ganja was growing at the grave of King Solomon, and in yet another reference to her ability to "relieve ignorance," Rastafarians consider her to be the "wisdom weed." They believe that the holy herb is the purest and most natural form of attaining communion with one's inner spiritual self; with their god, Jah; and with

Creation. Contrary to most who follow the Bible, Rastafarians assert that each individual and generation must gain and experience spiritual knowledge for themselves. They do not believe that one generation established all religious knowledge.

The Rastafarian religion and its love of ganja has spread all over the world through its music, reggae, and especially through the world's most famous reggae artist, Bob Marley. Because you can't keep a good herb down.

Ethiopia: Land of Lions and Zionists

Ethiopians founded the Zion Coptic Church, an offshoot of the Jamaican Rastafarian movement, in the 1970s. Perhaps it is best to understand their beliefs through the words of one of its late elders, Walter Wells.

The Coptic Church believes fully the teachings of the Bible, and as such we have our daily oblations, and offer our sacrifices, make by fire unto our God with chants and Psalms and spiritual hymns, lifting up holy hands and making melody in our hearts.

Herb is a Godly creation from the beginning of the world. It is known as the "Weed of Wisdom," "Angel's Food," the "Tree of Life," and even the "Wicked Old Ganja Tree." Its purpose in creation is as a fiery sacrifice to be offered to our Redeemer during oblations.

Ganja is not for commerce; yet because of the oppression of the people, it was raised up as the only liberator of the people and the only peacemaker among the entire generation. Ganja is the sacramental right of every man worldwide.[44]

CONCLUSION

May Her Spirit Heal Society

Why do you stay in prison, when the door is so wide open?

RUMI

We have witnessed that the great herb has a spirit, and that she is here to heal our spirits, as she has been doing the world over for thousands of years. She is a whole being and can heal our whole beings—mind, body, and spirit. She is the Emerald Trinity.

Just as marijuana medicine heals us personally on the spiritual level, it has the potential to heal our personal relationships, conflicts within society, and disputes throughout the globe. Reinvigorating "peace pipe" rituals can engender acceptance, compassion, and respect in communication and understanding between world governments and leaders. What could they accomplish with the courage to engage heart-to-heart instead of head-to-head?

Conflict is often rooted in patterns copied from generations of our family, hardened morals entrenched in us by society, and the ingrained habit of judging others. Prejudices and envy arise when we consider others as separate and different—and therefore inferior or superior to ourselves.

Robert Melamede, Ph.D., professor in, and former chairperson of, the biology department at the University of Colorado, said, "The extreme intolerance toward all forms of fuller expression can be traced to an operational deficit in the cannabinoid system."[1]

By showing us our distorted rationalizations, preconceived notions, and self-serving motives, ganja brings insight to our inner discord and contradictions. She advises us to answer our problems using our heart instead of our brains. She reminds us that the material world is an illusion and heaven is here and now. She paves the way for us to ponder our deepest spiritual questions: Who am I? How am I deceiving myself? Why am I here?

Cannabis can physically unpave unhealthy neural grooves that have been embedded by repetition throughout our lives. Been having that same old argument with your spouse and getting nowhere? Does it resemble arguments that your parents had? Smoking a little weed with your partner can help you find the real issue behind the conflict and a healthier way to communicate about it. Being high puts us into a more yin (receptive) mode of communication. We are more sensitive to nonverbal language. We can focus on the present with patience, truly listen to each other, and sense hidden feelings that drive repetitive rhetoric. We can give our full attention to each other instead of distractedly and disrespectfully forming our next response while they are still talking. Being a little stoned can invite compassion, calm, empathy, and respect into our interactions, and it helps us look past the usual defense systems that prevent the vulnerability and intimacy needed for quality communication.

Ultimately Mary Jane helps us realize that a conflict with another is mirrored by a conflict within ourselves. The greater spiritual lessons of life, like that we are all part of one organism, come to light, and how it is that attacking someone else is harming ourselves, caring for another is supporting ourselves, and even that taking care of ourselves supports those around us as well. When we become aware that we are all one, interpersonal conflicts fade away.

Spiritual practices are often criminalized or abandoned by societies during eras of materialism and authoritarianism, and they are replaced by enforced, rigid edicts of competition, punishment, separateness, racism, sexism, and suspicion of those who don't fit into an extremely narrow definition of normal. Corporate societies constantly bombard populations with subconscious messages like "money is the ultimate goal of life," "my people are better than your people," "nature must be destroyed for profit," "your profit must come at the expense of others," and "heaven/happiness comes only after death." Spending time alone, seeking silence, and personal spirituality are viewed with suspicion. A happy boss is more important than a happy family. Children are overwhelmed with ever-faster videos and computer games, busywork homework, gifted programs, continuous screen time, competitive organized sports, and activities that accelerate linear thought. This prepares them for a future of giving fifty to sixty hours a week of spiritless productivity to wealth-hoarding corporations. When do they develop feminine values like cooperation, connection with nature, creativity, and how to nurture themselves and others? Are they learning how to find inner peace?

I believe that the recent almost magnetic draw between marijuana and Western cultures represents an intrinsic human drive to move away from fundamentally dysfunctional patterns of interaction. When weed was reintroduced to the West in the 1960s, thanks to Vietnam veterans, an antiwar movement broke out. So did a movement to save the environment. Artists and musicians claimed greater roles in society. These very anticapitalistic movements soon became targets of a frightened government's propaganda and harassment until they almost disappeared by the '80s.

> *If the words "life, liberty, and the pursuit of happiness" don't include the right to experiment with your own consciousness, then the Declaration of Independence isn't worth the hemp it was written on.*
>
> TERENCE MCKENNA

Perhaps the current much wider spread of marijuana use will help our society move back in this direction. I can't help but think about how many people have benefitted from the medicinal effects of cannabis in the last five years. How many of them will experience that little miracle and advance to experimenting with her mind-altering properties? Will Mary Jane once again help humans evolve? Can we, as a society, release our intolerance of "other" and its accompanying systemic violence this time around? Mary Jane is certainly helping our medical system to evolve, and the rest of our crumbling social systems seem poised to follow. Can we rebuild a healthier, more balanced society? Can we replace senseless overproductivity with creativity? Advertising with art? Money with gifts? What would it look like, a society of people with a renewed sense of wonder and awe, reconnected to nature, and prone to fearless self-expression and personal pursuits?

Since she was churned in that Ocean of Milk oh so long ago, the Manna of the Gods has been trodden down, persecuted, and kidnapped ad nauseum by jealous "authorities," but they have never succeeded in keeping her down. A plant with magic crystals that grows like a weed, she has always been there for people and will continue to help us weather our own evolution. Although our current generations face a frightful future while the planet demonstrates her powers of destruction, Mary Jane will be there to help us through the great transition.

Like the seeds carried by the old merchant ships in case of shipwreck, if we keep her close, we will have food, material to rebuild, safe medicine to prevent and treat illness and injury, peace to fill our souls, a source of happiness in times of trouble, and a source of strength in times of grief. All of us have ancestors that used marijuana. All of us have ancestors that *were* marijuana. Her vast system of molecules and energy are found at the core of our beings. Indeed, they created the core of our beings. And because of this we are programmed for bliss.

Thank you for joining me in this journey to discover all the magic in marijuana medicine. It has been my life's work to collect this information, and now I have passed it on to you. May you invite the Emerald Trinity into your life and pass her on throughout the world so that we may all heal. May the following hymn from the *Rig Veda* help you connect with the spirit of the plant world.

Hymn to the Plants

Plants which as receptacles of light
were born three ages before the Gods,
I honor your myriad colors
and your seven hundred natures.
A hundred, oh Mothers, are your natures
and a thousand are your growths.
May you of a hundred powers
make whole what has been hurt.
Plants, as Mothers, as Goddesses, I address you.
May I gain the energy, the light, the sustenance,
your soul, you who are the human being.
Where the herbs are gathered together
like kings in an assembly,
there the doctor is called a sage,
who destroys evil,
and averts disease.
As they fell from Heaven, the plants said,
"The living soul we pervade,
that man will suffer no harm."
The Herbs which are in the kingdom of the Moon,
manifold with a hundred eyes,
I take you as the best of them,
for the fulfillment of wishes, as peace to the heart.
The plants which are queens of the Soma,
spread over all the Earth, generated by
the Lord of Prayer,
may your energies combine within this herb.

RIG VEDA, MANDALA 10, HYMN 97 (FROM *THE*
COMPLETE RIG VEDA, TRANSLATED BY RALPH
T. H. GRIFFITH, 1896. PUBLISHED BY CLASSIC
CENTURY WORKS, 2012)

APPENDIX

Phytocannabinoid Functions

All phytocannabinoids are formed from cannabigerolic acid (CBGA). CBGA decarboxlyates to CBG. In science CBGA is called the precursor to CBG. CBG is the biosynthetic precursor to all other phytocannabinoid acids, which then decarboxylate to various phytocannabinoids. In other words, CBGA is the first molecule synthesized by the plant. It then turns into CBG. CBG can then turn into any of the other cannabinoid acids, like THCA, CBDA, CBCA, or others. These cannabinoid acids then decarboxylate, through heat, light, or age, into phytocannabinoids like THC, CBD, CBC, or others. CBG is often referred to as the mother of all (phyto)cannabinoids, so I think of CBGA as the grandmother. I think of phytocannabinoid acids as daughters, and phytocannabinoids as granddaughters and great-granddaughters.

In chemistry, we represent these relationships with arrows like this: CBGA → CBG → THCA → THC → CBN. In this example, CBGA is the precursor to CBG which is the precursor to THCA, and so on. CBN would be a great-granddaughter.

Each form of every phytocannabinoid has a unique set of medicinal qualities. I have listed some of them in the pages that follow.

CANNABIGEROLIC ACID (CBGA), GRANDMOTHER OF ALL PHYTOCANNABINOIDS
CBGA → CBG

Analgesic

Antibacterial

Anti-inflammatory

Antiproliferative

CANNABIGEROL (CBG)
CBGA → CBG → ANY OTHER CANNABINOID ACID

Non-psychoactive

Analgesic

Antianxiety

Antibacterial

Anti-inflammatory

Antiproliferative

Antiseptic

Antitumor

Promotes bone growth

Reduces eye pressure

CANNABIDIOLIC ACID (CBDA)
CBGA → CBG → CBDA → CBD

Non-psychoactive

Found in raw leaf and flower

Anticancer

Anti-inflammatory

Antinausea

Antiproliferative

Antioxidant

Antipsychotic

Antitumor

Quells nausea and vomiting

CANNABIDIOL (CBD)
CBGA → CBG → CBDA → CBD

Non-psychoactive

Analgesic

Antianxiety

Antibacterial (potent against MRSA)

Anticancer

Potent anticonvulsant

Antidepressant

Antidiabetic

Potent anti-inflammatory

Anti-ischemic

Antinausea

Potent antioxidant

Antipsychotic

Antispasmodic

Antitumor

Reduces severity and frequency of autism

Biphasic (different doses cause different results)

Promotes bone growth

Alters gene expression of the ID1 gene

Boosts mitochondrial efficiency

Muscle relaxant

Prevents and aids neurodegenerative disorders

Stimulates neurogenesis

Neuroprotectant

Prevents and removes plaque and twisted proteins in the brain

Enhances sleep

Vasorelaxant

Stops vomiting

Antidote for overmedication with THC

Moderates the psychoactivity of THC

Balances increased heart rate induced by THC

Boosts endocannabinoids

Boosts the effects of other cannabinoids and all the other chemicals in the plant

CANNABIDIVARIN (CBDV)
CBGA → CBG → CBDVA → **CBDV**

Analgesic, especially for neuropathic pain and migraines

Antiepileptic

Anti-inflammatory

Alleviates autism symptoms including anxiety, seizures, addictive behavior, and mood disorders

Bone stimulant

CANNABICHROMENE (CBC)
CBGA → CBG → CBCA → **CBC**

Warning: CBC has caused hypothermia, sedation, and hypoactivity in mice. (A prayer for the tortured mice and the scientists who tortured them.)

Analgesic

Potent antianxiety

Anticancer

Antifungal

Anti-inflammatory

Antimicrobial

Antitumor

Promotes bone growth

Neuroprotective

Non-psychoactive

Boosts endocannabinoids

Believed to be 2.5 times stronger than THC

TETRAHYDROCANNABINOLIC ACID (THCA)
CBGA → CBG → **THCA** → THC

Non-psychoactive as found in raw leaf and flower

Anticancer

Anticonvulsant

Anti-inflammatory

Antinausea

Antineoplastic for noncancerous growths

Antioxidant

Antispasmodic

Antitumor

Immunomodulatory

Neuroprotective

Note: There are two forms, or isomers, of THC found in cannabis, Delta-8-tetrahydrocannabinol (Delta-8-THC) and Delta-9-tetrahydrocannabinol (Delta-9-THC).

DELTA-8-TETRAHYDROCANNABINOL (DELTA-8-THC)
CBGA → CBG → THCA → **DELTA-8-THC**

Warning: Because naturally occurring Delta-8-THC occurs in such trace amounts, most commercial Delta-8-THC is lab synthesized from CBD. It is only safe to consume if made from high-quality CBD and the caustic acids involved in the process are entirely eliminated from the finished product.

Psychoactive

Antinausea

DELTA-9-TETRAHYDROCANNABINOL (THC OR DELTA-9-THC)

CBGA → CBG → THCA → **DELTA-9-THC**

Psychoactive
Analgesic
Antianxiety
Anticancer
Antidepressant
Antidiabetic
Anti-inflammatory
Antinausea, stops vomiting
Potent antioxidant
Antitumor
Appetite stimulant
Biphasic (different doses cause different results)
Normalizes blood pressure
Stimulates creativity
Euphoriant
Reduces eye pressure

Accelerates heart rate (can lead to paranoia or anxiety in new users)
Dries mouth
Neuroprotective
Modulates neurotransmitters
Muscle relaxant
Perspective-altering
Can aggravate (but not cause) psychosis
Improves sensory perception
Induces sleep
Spirit-activating
Tissue protective
Boosts the effects of other cannabinoids and all the other chemicals in the plant

DELTA-9-TETRAHYDROCANNBIVARIN (THCV)

CBGA → CBG → THCVA → **THCV**

Analgesic
Antianxiety
Anticonvulsant
Antiemetic
Antiepileptic
Anti-inflammatory
Antinausea
Antioxidant
Appetite suppressant

Regulates blood sugar levels
Bone stimulant
Neuroprotective
Enhances serotonin receptors
Stimulating
Reduces tremors
Low dose suppresses THC
High dose enhances THC
Decreases time of THC activity

CANNABINOL (CBN)

CBGA → CBG →CBNA (OR THCA → THC) → **CBN**

Note: CBN can convert from CBNA or THC (with age)

Mildly psychoactive

Analgesic, bolstered by THC

Antibacterial (potent against MRSA)

Anticonvulsant

Antifungal

Antinausea

Antiseptic

Stimulates appetite

Regulates autoimmune issues

Regulates blood sugar

Promotes bone growth

Reduces eye pressure

Hypnotic

Relieves neuropathic pain

Sedative

Breakdown product of THC

Boosts psychoactivity of THC

Notes

CHAPTER 1.
CANNABINOIDS AND THE ENDOCANNABINOID SYSTEM

1. Anna Borsodi, Michael Bruchas, Girolamo Caló, Charles Chavkin, MacDonald J. Christie, Olivier Civelli, Mark Connor, et al., "Opioid Receptors in GtoPdb V.2023.1," *IUPHAR/BPS Guide to Pharmacology CITE* 1 (2023).

2. Leo Bear McGuinness, "DEA Awards Seventh Cannabis Cultivation License For Research Purposes," Analytical Cannabis website, August 22, 2022.

3. Alicia Wallace, "Patent No. 6,630,507: Why the U.S. Government Holds a Patent on Cannabis Plant Compounds," Denver Post website, August 28, 2016.

4. Aidan J. Hampson, Julius Axelrod, and Maurizio Grimaldi, Cannabinoids as antioxidants and neuroprotectants, US patent US6630507B1, filed April 21, 1999, and granted October 7, 2003.

5. Sandra Young, "Marijuana Stops Child's Severe Seizures," CNN website, August 7, 2013.

6. Markus Kathmann, Karsten Flau, Agnes Redmer, Christian Tränkle, and Eberhard Schlicker, "Cannabidiol Is an Allosteric Modulator at Mu- and Delta-opioid Receptors," *Naunyn Schmiedeberg's Archives of Pharmacology* 372, no. 5 (February 2006): 354–61.

7. Ethan B. Russo, "Clinical Endocannabinoid Deficiency (CECD): Can This Concept Explain Therapeutic Benefits of Cannabis in Migraine, Fibromyalgia, Irritable Bowel Syndrome and Other Treatment-resistant Conditions?" *Neuro Endocrinology Letters* 29, no. 2 (April 2008): 192–200.

8. Jeremy Gungabeesoon, "Liverwort as an Alternative to Medical Cannabis,"

Science in the News, a blog of Harvard University Graduate School of Arts and Sciences, November 1, 2018.

CHAPTER 2.
TRUTH AND RECONCILIATION: MOVING BEYOND PROPAGANDA AND PERSECUTION

1. "A Brief History of Medical Cannabis in the United States," Alternative Compassion Services website, accessed July 14, 2023.

2. Quoted in "Henry Ford's Hemp Cars," The Meaning of Water website, October 3, 2020.

3. Gooey Rabinski, "Meet the Man Responsible for Marijuana Prohibition," Mass Roots website, accessed August 15, 2021.

4. Rabinski, "Meet the Man Responsible for Marijuana Prohibition."

5. Dialogue as quoted in Richard J. Bonnie and Charles H. Whitebread, "The Forbidden Fruit and the Tree of Knowledge: An Inquiry into the Legal History of American Marijuana Prohibition," *Virginia Law Review* 56, no. 6 (1970).

6. Dan Baum, "Legalize It All," *Harper's*, April 2016.

7. The Leadership Conference Education Fund, "End Drug War, Says Jimmy Carter and Members of Congress," Civil Rights website, June 17, 2011.

8. Christopher Ingraham, "Trump's Pick for Attorney General: 'Good People Don't Smoke Marijuana,'" *Washington Post*, November 18, 2016.

9. Mark Frauenfelder, "Harvard Psychiatrist on David Brooks' Pot Column: 'His Ignorance about This Subject Is Vast,'" Boing Boing website, January 8, 2014.

10. Lester Grinspoon, "A Cannabis Odyssey: To Smoke or Not to Smoke," Marijuana-Users website under the Read tab, April 20, 2009.

11. Sanjay Gupta, "Why I Changed My Mind on Weed," CNN website, August 8, 2013.

12. Christine Milentis, "IACM 2019 Highlights: Defending Doctor's Rights Across the Globe," Society of Cannabis Clinicians website, December 19, 2019.

13. "Emerging Clinical Applications of Cannabis," *O'Shaughnessy's: The Journal of Cannabis in Clinical Practice* (Winter/Spring 2007), as cited in Julie Holland, *The Pot Book* (Rochester, VT.: Park Street Press, 2010).

14. David F. Duncan, "Lifetime Prevalence of 'Amotivational Syndrome' Among Users and Non-users of Hashish," *Psychology of Addictive Behaviors* 1, no. 2 (1987): 114–19.

15. Roy Richard Grinker, "In Retrospect: The Five Lives of the Psychiatry Manual," *Nature* 468 (November 10, 2010): 168–69.

16. Joseph Maroon and Jeff Bost, "Review of the Neurological Benefits of Phytocannabinoids," *Surgical Neurology International* 9 (2018): 91.

17. Ann Kreilkamp, "Dr. Lester Grinspoon on Marijuana: 'I Finally Decided in 1973 that I Would Start Using It, and I've Been Using It Ever Since,'" Exopermaculture website, January 10, 2014.

18. Julie Holland, *The Pot Book* (Rochester, VT.: Park Street Press, 2010), 385.

19. Martijn Schirp, "Carl Sagan's Profound Essay on Why Cannabis Consciousness Is Desperately Needed in This Mad and Dangerous World," High Existence website, February 3, 2020.

20. Luka Dobovišek, Metka Novak, Fran Krstanović, Polonca Ferk, Simona Borštnar, Tamara Lah Turnšek, and Nataša Debeljak, "Cannabidiol Increases Potency of Tamoxifen in Inhibiting Breast Cancer Cell Viability," *Cancer Research* 80, no. 4 suppl. (2020): P3-05-11.

21. "Cannabis Drug Interactions and Side-Effects with Dr. Franjo Grotenherman," Cannabis Radio website, November 2019.

22. Mahra Nourbakhsh, Angela Miller, Jeff Gofton, Graaham Jones, Bamidele Adeagbo, "Cannabinoid Hyperemesis Syndrome: Reports of Fatal Cases," *Journal of Forensic Sciences* 64, issue 1 (January 2019): 270–74.

23. Cecilia J. Sorensen, Kristen DeSanto, Laura Borgelt, Kristina T. Phillips, and Andrew A. Monte, "Cannabinoid Hyperemesis Syndrome: Diagnosis, Pathophysiology, and Treatment—A Systematic Review," *Journal of Medical Toxicology* 13, no. 1 (2017): 71–87.

24. Stephen E. Nicolson, Lex Denysenko, J. Loretta Mulcare, Jose P. Vito, and Brenda Chabon, "Cannabinoid Hyperemesis Syndrome: A Case Series and Review of Previous Reports," *Psychosomatics* 53, no. 3 (May–June 2012): 212–19.

25. Ethan B. Russo, Chris Spooner, Len May, Ryan Leslie, and Venetia L. Whiteley, "Cannabinoid Hyperemesis Syndrome Survey and Genomic Investigation," *Cannabis and Cannabinoid Research* 7, no. 3 (2022): 336–44.

26. Carl L. Hart, Wilfred van Gorp, Margaret Haney, Richard W. Foltin, and Marian W. Fischman, "Effects of Acute Smoked Marijuana on Complex Cognitive Performance," *Neuropsychopharmacology* 25, no. 5 (November 2001): 757–65.

27. Holland, *The Pot Book,* 370.

CHAPTER 3.
WHOLE PLANT MEDICINE

1. For information about alpha-pinene, limonene, and caryophyllene's antiviral properties, especially those specific to COVID, see Destinney Cox-Georgian, Niveditha Ramadoss, Chanthu Dona, and Chhandak Basu, "Therapeutic and Medicinal Uses of Terpenes," *Medicinal Plants,* November 12, 2019, 333–59.
2. Natasha R. Ryz, David J. Remillard, and Ethan B. Russo, "Cannabis Roots: A Traditional Therapy with Future Potential for Treating Inflammation and Pain," *Cannabis and Cannabinoid Research* 2, no. 1 (2017): 210–16.

CHAPTER 4.
WEED FOR MENTAL WELLNESS

1. Joan Bello, *The Benefits of Marijuana: Physical, Psychological, and Spiritual* (Susquehanna, PA.: Lifeservices Press, 2008), 49.
2. Lester Grinspoon, "A Cannabis Odyssey: To Smoke or Not to Smoke," Marijuana-Users website under the Read tab, April 20, 2009.
3. Among myriad others, see, for example: Maya J. Lambiase, Laura D. Kubzansky, and Rebecca C. Thurston, "Positive Psychological Health and Stroke Risk: The Benefits of Emotional Vitality," *Health Psychology* 34 (October 2015): 1043–46; Ed Diener and Robert Biswas-Diener, *Happiness: Unlocking the Mysteries of Psychological Wealth* (Hoboken, NJ: Wiley-Blackwell, 2008); Min Li, Xiao-Wei Zhang, Wen-Shang Hou, and Zhen-YuTang, "Impact of Depression on Incident Stroke: A Meta-analysis," *International Journal of Cardiology* 180 (February 2015): 103–10; Robert M. Carney and Kenneth E. Freedland, "Depression and Coronary Heart Disease," *National Review of Cardiology* 14 (2017): 145–55.
4. See Natan Kellermann, "Epigenetic transmission of Holocaust Trauma: Can nightmares be inherited?" *Israel Journal of Psychiatry and Related Sciences* 50, no. 1 (2013): 33–39.
5. Bello, *Benefits of Marijuana,* 37–39.
6. See the Vanderbuilt University Medical Center website, search for "Patel lab."
7. Michael H. Bloch, Christy Green, Stephen A. Kichuk, Philip A. Dombrowski, Suzanne Wasylink, Eileen Billingslea, Angeli Landeros-Weisenberger, et al., "Long-term Outcome in Adults with Obsessive-Compulsive Disorder," *Depression and Anxiety* 30 (2013): 716–22.

8. Dakota Mauzay, Emily M. LaFrance, and Carrie Cuttler, "Acute Effects of Cannabis on Symptoms of Obsessive-Compulsive Disorder," *Journal of Affective Disorders* 279 (2021): 158–63.

9. Felipe V. Gomes, Plinio C. Casarotto, Leonardo B. M. Resstel, and Francisco Guimarães, "Facilitation of CB1 Receptor-mediated Neurotransmission Decreases Marble Burying Behavior in Mice," *Progress in Neuro-Psychopharmacology and Biological Psychiatry* 35, no. 2, (2011): 434–38.

10. "What is an Autistic Savant?" on the Applied Behavior Analysis Edu (organization) website, accessed July 19, 2023.

11. Bonni Goldstein, *Cannabis Revealed: How the World's Most Misunderstood Plant Is Healing Everything from Chronic Pain to Epilepsy,* (self-published, 2016), 145.

12. Mauro Maccarrone, Silvia Rossi, Monica Bari, Valentina De Chiara, Cinzia Rapino, Alessandra Musella, Giorgio Bernardi, Claudia Bagni, Diego Centonze. "Abnormal mGlu 5 Receptor/Encocannbinoid Coupling in Mice Lacking FMRP and BC1 RNA." *Neuropsychopharmacology* 35 no. 7 (2010): 1500–09; Kwang-Mook Jung, et al., "Uncoupling of the Endocanabinoid Signaling Complex in a Mouse Model of Fragile X Syndrome," *Nature Communications* 3 (2012): 1080.

13. Dana Barchel, Orit Stolar, Tal De-Haan, Tomer Ziv-Baran, Naama Saban, Danny Or Fuchs, Gideon Koren, and Matithu Berkovitz, "Oral Cannabidiol Use in Children with Autism Spectrum Disorder to Treat Related Symptoms and Comorbidities," *Frontiers in Pharmacology* 9 (January 2019): 1521.

14. Lihi Bar-Lev Schleider, Raphael Mechoulam, Naama Saban, Gal Meiri, and Victor Novack, "Real Life Experience of Medical Cannabis Treatment in Autism: Analysis of Safety and Efficacy," *Scientific Reports* 9, no. 1 (January 2019): 200.

15. See Mariano Garcia de Palau, "Cannabinoids and Autism Spectrum Disorder," on the Fundación Canna website, accessed July 19, 2023.

16. Marian Fry, cannabis clinician, from a survey printed in *O'Shaughnessy's: The Journal of Cannabis in Clinical Practice.*

17. Quoted in Mike Colagrossi, "How Non-industrial Cultures View Mental Illness," Big Think website, November 5, 2018.

18. Stephanie Marohn, *The Natural Medicine Guide to Schizophrenia* (Newburyport, MA: Hampton Road Publishing Co., 2003), 178–89, as quoted on Jayson Gaddis, "The Shamanic View of Mental Illness," Uplift Connect website, February 26, 2019.

19. W. D. Fabian, Jr. and S. M. Fishkin, "Psychological Absorption: Affect Investment in Marijuana Intoxication," *Journal of Nervous and Mental Disease* 179, no. 1 (January 1991): 39–43.

20. "Statistics on Stimulant Use," PBS Frontline website, accessed July 19, 2023.

21. Cayla Clark, "What Are the Long Term Effects of Adderall & Methamphetamine?" Guardian Recovery Network website, April 23, 2020.

22. NIDA, "What Is the Scope of Methamphetamine Misuse in the United States?" National Institute on Drug Abuse (NIDA) website, February 13, 2023.

23. Callie Rushton, "Jim Carrey explains Depression in the Best Way I've ever Heard" Elephant Journal website, December 1, 2017.

24. Peter R. Breggin, "Suicidality, Violence and Mania Caused by Selective Serotonin Reuptake Inhibitors (SSRIs): A Review and Analysis," *International Journal of Risk & Safety in Medicine* 16 (2003/2004): 31–49.

25. Jeanne Stolzer, "The Systemic Correlation Between Psychiatric Medications and Unprovoked Mass Murder in America," *New Male Studies: An International Journal* 2, no. 2, (2013): 9–23.

26. Cristina Benito, Estefania Nunez, Rosa M. Tolon, Erica J. Carrier, Alberto Rabano, Cecilia J. Hillard, and Julian Romero, "Cannabinoid CB2 Receptors and Fatty Acid Amide Hydrolase Are Selectively Overexpressed in Neuritic Plaque-associated Glia in Alzheimer's Disease Brains," *Journal of Neuroscience* 23 (2003): 11136–41.

27. Kwakye Peprah and Suzanne McCormack, "Medical Cannabis for the Treatment of Dementia: A Review of Clinical Effectiveness and Guidelines [Internet]," Ottawa (ON): Canadian Agency for Drugs and Technologies in Health, July 17, 2019.

28. Peprah and McCormack, "Medical Cannabis for the Treatment of Dementia."

29. Jeffrey Hergenrather, personal interview with the author, March 2018.

30. Ethan B. Russo, "Cannabis Therapeutics and the Future of Neurology," *Frontiers of Integrative Neuroscience* 12 (2018); Christine Milentis, "IACM 2019 Highlights: Defending Doctors' Rights Across the Globe," Society of Cannabis Clinicians website, December 19, 2019.

31. L. J. Thompson and R. C. Proctor, "The Use of Pyrahexyl in the Treatment of Alcoholic and Drug Withdrawal Conditions," *North Carolina Medical Journal* 14, no. 10 (1953): 520–23.

32. Edward M. Brecher and the Editors of *Consumer Reports Magazine,* "The Consumers Union Report on Licit and Illicit Drugs", published in 1972, available on the Drug Library website.

33. W. Mackworth Young, Report of the Indian Hemp Drugs Commission 1893–94, *Volume 1,* available on the Hardinge Simpole website (in association with the National Library of Scotland).

34. Tod Hiro Mikuriya, "Cannabis as A Substitute for Alcohol," *Journal of Cannabis Therapeutics* 4, no. 1 (2004).

35. University of British Columbia, "Marijuana Could Help Treat Drug Addiction, Mental Health, Study Suggests," Science Daily website, November 16, 2016.

36. Mikuriya, "Cannabis as A Substitute for Alcohol."

37. Harvard Health Publishing, "Treating Opiate Addiction Part I: Detoxification and Maintenance," Harvard Health website, June 27, 2019.

38. Marcus A. Bachhuber, Brendan Saloner, Chinazo O. Cunningham, and Colleen L. Barry, "Medical Cannabis Laws and Opioid Analgesic Overdose Mortality in the United States, 1999–2010." *JAMA Internal Medicine* 174, no. 10 (2014): 1668–73.

39. Adam Schmidt, "Can Marijuana Help the Country Deal with the Opioid Crisis?" Clear Choice Cannabis website, July 4, 2018.

40. Eric Killelea, "How Medical Marijuana Could Help End the Opioid Epidemic," Rolling Stone website, March 29, 2017.

41. Lester Grinspoon and James B. Bakalar, *Marihuana: The Forbidden Medicine* (New Haven, CT: Yale University Press, 1993).

CHAPTER 5.
PHYSICAL SYSTEMS AND CONDITIONS THAT BENEFIT FROM CANNABIS

1. David M. Fergusson, L. John Horwood, and Kate Northstone, "Maternal Use of Cannabis and Pregnancy Outcome," *BJOG: An International Journal of Obstetrics & Gynaecology* 109 (2002): 21–27.

2. Two resources are the American Cannabis Nurses Association and Canna Mommy websites.

3. J. Zias, "Cannabis as an Effective Medication in Antiquity: The Anthropological Evidence," presented at The Archaeology of Death in the Near East International Conference held at Victoria University of Manchester, Fallowfiled Campus, December 16–19, 1992, available at the Deutsches Archaologisches Institute website.

4. Steve Connor, "Remains Found of Ancient Dope Smoker: Cannabis Used as Painkiller in Fourth Century," *Independent,* May 20, 1993.

5. Ethan B. Russo, "Cannabis Treatments in Obstetrics and Gynecology," *Journal of Cannabis Therapeutics* 2, nos. 3–4 (June 2002): 5–35.

6. Russo, "Cannabis Treatments in Obstetrics and Gynecology."

7. Russo, "Cannabis Treatments in Obstetrics and Gynecology."

8. Russo, "Cannabis Treatments in Obstetrics and Gynecology."

9. Alexander Christison, "On the Natural History, Action, and Uses of Indian Hemp." *Monthly Journal of Medical Science* 4, no. 20 (1851): 117–121.

10. As quoted in Russo, "Cannabis Treatments in Obstetrics and Gynecology."

11. Maud Grieve, *A Modern Herbal* (New York: Dover, 1971 [first published in 1931]).

12. Melanie C. Dreher, "Maternal–Child Health and Ganja in Jamaica," *Studies in Third World Societies* 30 (December 1984). PDF available from the CIFAS website (Comitas Institute for Anthropological Study) under the Research tab.

13. Jeffrey Hergenrather, personal interview with the author, March 2019.

14. Christine Milentis, "IACM 2019 Highlights: Defending Doctors' Rights Across the Globe," Society of Cannabis Clinicians website, December 19, 2019.

15. Wei-Ni Lin Curry, "Hyperemesis Gravidarum and Clinical Cannabis: To Eat or Not to Eat?" published simultaneously in *Journal of Cannabis Therapeutics* 2, no. 3/4 (2002): 63–83 and in Ethan Russo, Melanie Dreher, and Mary Lynn Mathre, *Women and Cannabis: Medicine, Science, and Sociology* (New York: Haworth Integrative Healing Press, 2002), 63–83.

16. A. E. Munson, L. S. Harris, M. A. Friedman, W. L. Dewey, and R. A. Carchman, "Antineoplastic Activity of Cannabinoids," *Journal of the National Cancer Institute* 55, no. 3 (September 1975): 597–602.

17. Michael Taillard, "Cannabis Can Cure Many Forms of Cancer," Cure Your Own Cancer website under the Scientific Studies tab.

18. C. Sanchez, I. Galve-Roperh, C. Canova, P. Brachet, and M. Guzman, "Delta-9-tetrahydrocannabinol induces apoptosis in C6 glioma cells," *FEBS Letters* 436, no. 1 (September 1998): 6–10.

19. Maria M. Medveczky, Tracy A. Sherwood, Thomas W. Klein, Herman Friedman, and Peter G. Medveczky, "Delta-9 Tetrahydrocannabinol (THC) Inhibits Lytic Replication of Gamma Oncogenic Herpesviruses in vitro," *BMC Med* 2 (2004): 34.

20. American Association for Cancer Research, "Marijuana Cuts Lung Cancer Tumor Growth in Half, Study Shows," Science Daily website, April 17, 2007; M. Guzmán, M. J. Duarte, C. Blázquez, J. Ravina, M. C. Rosa, I. Galve-Roperh, C. Sánchez, G. Velasco, and L. González-Feria, "A Pilot Clinical Study of Delta-9-tetrahydrocannabinol in Patients with Recurrent Glioblastoma Multiforme," *British Journal of Cancer* 95 (2006): 197–203.

21. Robin Wilkey, "Marijuana and Cancer: Scientists Find Cannabis Compound Stops Metastasis in Aggressive Cancers," Huffpost website, September 19, 2012.

22. NORML, "National Institutes of Cancer Website Recognizes Cancer-killing Properties of Cannabinoids," NORML website, March 31, 2011.

23. "Dr. William Courtney Calls Child 'A Miracle Baby,'" Cure Your Own Cancer website.

24. Bo Wang, Anna Kovalchuk, Dongping Li, Rocio Rodriguez-Juarez, Yaroslav Ilnytskyy, Igor Kovalchuk, and Olga Kovalchuk, "In Search of Preventative Strategies: Novel Anti-Inflammatory High-CBD Cannabis Sativa Extracts Modulate ACE2 Expression in COVID-19 Gateway Tissues," *Aging* 12, no. 22 (November 2020): 22425–44.

25. Juan L. Rodriguez, Joseph A. Lopez, and J. Jordan Steel, "Involvement of the Endocannabinoid System in the Inhibition of Sindbis Virus Replication: A Preliminary Study," *Journal of Cannabis Research* 3, no. 10 (2021).

26. Long Chi Nguyen, Dongbo Yang, Vlad Nicolaescu, Thomas J. Best, Takashi Ohtsuki, Shao-Nong Chen, J. Brent Friesen et al., "Cannabidiol Inhibits SARS-CoV-2 Replication and Promotes the Host Innate Immune Response," preprint March 10, 2021; updated peer-reviewed version of this study is Long Chi Nguyen, Dongbo Yang, Vlad Nicolaescu, Thomas J. Best, Haley Gula, Divyasha Saxena, Jon D. Gabbard, et al., "Cannabidiol inhibits SARS-CoV-2 Replication through Induction of the Host ER Stress and Innate Immune Responses," *Science Advances* 8, no. 8 (February 2022).

27. Monica R. Loizzo, Antoine M. Saab, Rosa Tundis, Giancarlo A. Statti, Francesco Menichini, Ilaria Lampronti, Roberto Gambari, Jindrich Cinatl, and Hans Wilhelm Doerr, "Phytochemical Analysis and in vitro Antiviral Activities of the Essential Oils of Seven Lebanon Species," *Chemistry & Biodiversity* 5, no. 3 (2008): 461–70.

28. Chandra Shekhar Nautiyal, Puneet Singh Chauhan, and Yeshwant Laxman Nene, "Medicinal Smoke Reduces Airborne Bacteria," *Journal of Ethnopharmacology* 114, no. 3 (December 2007): 446–51.

29. Seegehalli M. Anil, Nurit Shalev, Ajjampura C. Vinayaka, Stalin Nadarajan, Dvora Namdar, Eduard Belausov, Irit Shoval, Karthik Ananth Mani, Guy Mechrez, and Hinanit Koltai, "Cannabis Compounds Exhibit Anti-inflammatory Activity in vitro in COVID-19-related Inflammation in Lung Epithelial Cells and Pro-inflammatory Activity in Macrophages," *Scientific Reports* 11, article 1462 (2021).

30. Hasan K. Siddiqi, Peter Libby, and Paul M. Ridker, "COVID-19—A Vascular Disease," *Trends in Cardiovascular Medicine* 31, no. 1 (January 2021): 1–5.

31. Anil et al., "Cannabis Compounds Exhibit Anti-inflammatory Activity in vitro in COVID-19-related Inflammation in Lung Epithelial Cells and Pro-inflammatory Activity in Macrophages."

32. Benjamin T. Bradley and Andrew Bryan, "Emerging Respiratory Infections: The Infectious Disease Pathology of SARS, MERS, Pandemic Influenza, and Legionella," *Seminars in Diagnostic Pathology* 36, no. 3 (May 2019): 152–59.

33. Ana Sandoiu, "COVID-19 and the Brain: What Do We Know So Far?" Medical News Today website, January 25, 2021.

34. Sandoiu, "COVID-19 and the Brain: What Do We Know So Far?"

35. William A. Haseltine, "Covid-19: Long Term Brain Injury," Forbes website, March 14, 2022.

36. Eric Song, Ce Zhang, Benjamin Israelow, Alice Lu-Culligan, Alba Vieites Prado, Sophie Skriabine, Peiwen Lu, et al., "Neuroinvasion of SARS-CoV-2 in Human and Mouse Brain," *Journal of Experimental Medicine* 218, no. 3 (March 2021).

37. Wendy Corona, "New Study Shows COVID-19 Could Hide In Your Brain and Reactivate Down the Road," WSBTV website, January 20, 2021.

38. Jennifer Abbasi, "Even Mild COVID-19 May Change the Brain," *Journal of the American Medical Association* 327, no. 14 (2022): 1321–22.

39. Maxime Taquet, John R. Geddes, Masud Husain, Sierra Luciano, and Paul J. Harrison, "6-Month Neurological and Psychiatric Outcomes in 236,379 Survivors of COVID-19: A Retrospective Cohort Study Using Electronic Health Records," *The Lancet Psychiatry* 8, no. 5 (2021): 416–27.

CHAPTER 6.
TYPES OF MARIJUANA MEDICINE

1. Fred Gardner, "UCLA Lab Reports Surprising Results at ICRS Meeting: Smoking Cannabis Does Not Cause Cancer of Lung or Upper Airways, Tashkin Finds; Data Suggest Possible Protective Effect," *O'Shaughnessy's: The Journal of Cannabis in Clinical Practice* (Autumn 2005).

CHAPTER 8.
DEVELOPING A CANNABIS THERAPY PLAN

1. Project CBD, "The CBD User's Manual," Elm City Wellness website (reprinted with permission from Project CBD), March 13, 2018.

CHAPTER 9.
HOW TO MAKE MEDICINE WITH MARIJUANA

1. Chandra Shekhar Nautiyal, Puneet Singh Chauhan, and Yeshwant Laxman Nene, "Medicinal Smoke Reduces Airborne Bacteria," *Journal of Ethnopharmacology* 114, no. 3 (December 2007): 446–51.

CHAPTER 10.
THE SPIRIT OF GANJA AROUND THE WORLD

1. Quoted in Chris Bennett, *Cannabis and the Soma Solution* (Walterville, Oregon: Trine Day, 2010), 50.
2. Chris Bennett, "Kaneh Bosm: Cannabis in the Old Testament," Cannabis Culture website, May 1, 1996.
3. Walter Houston Clark, "Drug cult," Britannica website, July 24, 1998.
4. Personal correspondence with Chris Bennett.
5. I. L. Finkel, "A New Piece of Libanomancy," *Archiv für Orientforschung* 29 (1983): 50–57.
6. Joshua J. Mark, "The Myth of Etana," World History website, March 2, 2011.
7. Albert Hofmann, Christian Ratsch, and Richard Schultes, *Plants of the Gods: Their Sacred, Healing, and Hallucinogenic Powers* (Rochester, VT: Healing Arts Press, 1992).
8. Edward M. Brecher and the Editors of Consumer Reports, *Licit and Illicit Drugs: The Consumers Union Report on Narcotics, Stimulants, Depressants, Inhalants, Hallucinogens, and Marijuana, Including Caffeine, Nicotine, and Alcohol* (New York: Little, Brown & Co., 1973).
9. Herodotus, *The History of Herotodus,* book 4, verses 74–75, available on the Gutenberg website.
10. Simon Worrall, "Amazon Warriors Did Indeed Fight and Die Like Men," National Geographic website, October 28, 2014.
11. David Harding, "Two Solid Gold Bongs, Thought to be 2,400 Years Old, Discovered in Russia," NY Daily News website, May 30, 2015.
12. Bennett, *Cannabis and the Soma Solution,* 352, citing Polish anthropologist Sula Benet.
13. Chris Bennett, *Liber 420: Cannabis, Magickal Herbs and the Occult* (Walterville, Oregon: Trine Day, 2018).

14. Mircea Eliade, *A History of Religious Ideas: From the Stone Age to the Eleusinian Mysteries,* vol. 1 (Chicago: University of Chicago Press, 1981): 211–12.

15. *Yasna* 9:13, available on the Avesta (org) website, under the Yasna link.

16. *Yasna* 9:2.

17. *Yasna* 9:17.

18. Chris Bennett, "The Herb of the Magi: Zoroaster's Good Narcotic," Cannabis Culture website, October 1, 2019.

19. Bennett, "The Herb of the Magi: Zoroaster's Good Narcotic."

20. Bennett, *Cannabis and the Soma Solution,* 108–16.

21. Diana Stein, "Winged Disks and Sacred Trees at Nuzi: An Altered Perspective on Two Imperial Motifs," *Studies on the Civilization and Culture of Nuzi and the Hurrians* 18 (2009): 573–603.

22. Meng Ren, Zihua Tang, Xinhua Wu, Robert Spengler, Hongen Jiang, Yimin Yang, and Nicole Boivin, "The Origins of Cannabis Smoking: Chemical Residue Evidence from the First Millennium BCE in the Pamirs," *Science Advances* 5, no. 6 (June 2019).

23. Evan Hadingham, "The Mummies of Xinjiang," Discover Magazine online, April 1, 1994.

24. Quoted in David N. Keightley, *The Origins of Chinese Civilization* (Berkeley: University of California Press, 1983), 32.

25. Benjamin Schwartz, *The World of Thought in Ancient China* (Cambridge: Harvard University Press, 1985), 36.

26. Quoted in Joseph Needham, *Science and Civilisation in China,* vol. 2 (Cambridge, UK: Cambridge University Press, 1974), 151.

27. Cannalore, "Uncle Sam Breeds Hemp, 1901," The Canna Chronicles website, May 25, 2018.

28. Jon Mitchell, "Cannabis—The Fabric of Japan," *The Japan Times,* accessed August 22, 2021.

29. Chris Bennett, *Cannabis: Lost Sacrament of the Ancient World* (Walterville, Oregon: Keneh Press, 2023), 11.

30. Ezekiel 27:19 as quoted in Bennett, "Kaneh Bosm: Cannabis in the Old Testament."

31. Sula Benet, "Early Diffusions and Folk Uses of Hemp," reprinted in Vera Rubin, *Cannabis and Culture* (Berlin, Germany: Mouton de Gruyter, 1975).

32. Chris Bennett, "Cannabis and the Christ: Jesus Used Marijuana," Cannabis Culture website, January 2, 1998.

33. James M. Campbell, "Note on the Religion of Hemp," in W. Mackworth Young, *Report of the Indian Hemp Drugs Commission 1893–94*, available on the Hardinge Simpole website (in association with the National Library of Scotland).

34. Young, *Report of the Indian Hemp Drugs Commission 1893–94.*

35. Mahanirvana Tantra 5:5–7, quoted in Michael R. Aldrich, "Tantric Cannabis Use in India," *Journal of Psychedelic Drugs* 9, no. 3 (1977): 227–33.

36. Tod Hiro Mikuriya, *Marijuana Medical Papers 1839–1972* (Oakland, CA: Medi-Comp Press, 1973).

37. Mohammad Hassan Ibn-Chirazi, thirteenth-century account as appears in Bennett, *Liber 420: Cannabis, Magickal Herbs and the Occult.*

38. Quoted in Paul Lovejoy, Jordan Goodman, and Andrew Sherratt, *Consuming Habits: Global and Historical Perspectives on How Cultures Define Drugs* (Abingdon, U.K.: Routledge, 2007).

39. Dymock, 1890, as quoted in Bennett, *Cannabis and the Soma Solution*, 529.

40. Franz Rosenthal, *The Herb: Hashish versus Medieval Muslim Society* (Leiden: E. J. Bill, 1971), 41.

41. Chris Bennett, "The Mother Plant of the Goddess Cannabis," Cannabis Culture website, May 31, 2019, citing William Emboden, *Narcotic Plants* (New York: MacMillan, 1972), and Rosenthal, *The Herb: Hashish versus Medieval Muslim Society.*

42. Chris Bennett, "Hashish and Other Psychoactive Substances in Islam," Cannabis Culture website, November 22, 2018.

43. Chris Duvall, *The African Roots of Marijuana* (Durham, NC: Duke University Press, 2019).

44. John Brown and the Ethiopian Zion Coptic Church, *Marijuana and the Bible* (self-published: Createspace, 2012).

CONCLUSION.
MAY HER SPIRIT HEAL SOCIETY

1. Quoted in Joan Bello, *Benefits of Marijuana: The Physical, Psychological and Spiritual* (Susquehanna, PA: Lifeservices Press, 2008).

Index